T0267482

PENGUIN LIFE

SOOTHE

Nahid de Belgeonne is a Somatic Movement Educator and founder of The Human Method, a radical relearning system that works to harmonize the mind and body intelligently—dynamically transforming the health of everyone, from exhausted and burned-out highfliers, A-list celebrities and athletes, right through to clients who are recovering from illness, injury, sleep issues, stress, and anxiety. She runs an online clinic working with clients privately and on retreat. Nahid is a Londoner who now lives by the sea with her husband and three Boston terriers.

The Soothe Group Program is an online nervous-system reset to accompany the book, with on-demand classes and regular Q&A sessions. All the lessons in the book are covered, as well as other deep practices to help you reset your nervous system.

soothe

Restoring Your Nervous
System from Stress, Anxiety,
Burnout, and Trauma

Nahid de Belgeonne

life

Neither the publisher nor the author is engaged in rendering professional advice
or services to the individual reader. The ideas, procedures, and suggestions contained
in this book are not intended as a substitute for consulting with your physician.
All matters regarding your health require medical supervision. Neither the
author nor the publisher shall be liable or responsible for any loss or damage
allegedly arising from any information or suggestion in this book.

For Rudy de Belgeonne,
the one who soothes my soul

When the world tells you to shrink, expand.

Elaine Welteroth, *More Than Enough*

Contents

Introduction

Knowledge comes from our senses and if we extend our
senses then we will consequently extend our knowledge.
Neil Harbisson, "Extraordinary Senses: The Cyborg
Who Hears in Colour," *Outlook* podcast

Soothe: To gently calm, reduce pain or discomfort,
relieve, or ease.

I grew up in a house full of stress, unhappiness, and worry.
No one meant for that to happen, but it did. I learned to
suppress my true feelings because they were inconvenient,
both to me and to others, who were tightly bound to their
own suffering. For as long as I can remember, my feelings
were overwhelming because I had no place to put them.

My parents came to the UK in the 1960s from Bang-
ladesh and the experience was, by all accounts, exciting,
bold, and courageous, but also cold, unknown, isolating, and
sometimes menacing. They had the pressures of starting a
family in a different country and culture, away from their
extended community and without the safety net of that
support, as well as holding down demanding jobs. I was
born and brought up in multicultural London, which meant

there was easy social mixing between different people; but growing up in a volatile house with strict rules, angry words, and a bias toward men meant that my understanding of family life was combative and unhappy. There was always tension hanging in the air. My father left us to work abroad for a while and it was decided it would be best for the children, and probably for my mother, that we stayed at school and went to visit him during the holidays. That abandonment was never really spoken about. As often happens when you have one parent who carries the weight of bringing up the family, you tend not to talk about the things that are bothering you, because you don't want to add to their suffering. When your caregivers haven't learned how to soothe or comfort themselves, they can't pass on to you these valuable skills.

On a purely sensory level, I understood that movement helped to dissipate my feelings. I loved sports at school and I particularly enjoyed solo activities over team ones, to better quiet my mind. When I was physically engaged, I could shift my focus from my noisy head to the sensations of my body. The feelings of my body moving were so fully absorbing that I forgot to worry about all the things that might happen one day. I started running when I wanted to leave home; kickboxing when I wanted to leave my first husband; yoga when I left a highly paid but stressful job, with no plans. I also smoked weed to dampen my anxiety, because the effects of movement didn't last beyond the afterglow of the activity itself. I was looking for anything that would enable me to stop thinking, because my thoughts caused me mental anguish. I held two beliefs that only now, in hindsight, do I recognize: I believed that my feelings made me weak, and that resting would thwart my forward momentum. These beliefs formed me in adulthood.

On the outside, I appeared successful and easygoing. On the inside, everything that I achieved came at a cost to my mental and physical health. I routinely pushed myself through tiredness and illness. Over the years I suffered from chronic anxiety, bouts of panic, neuralgia, and urticaria, and I almost died from a burst appendix because I didn't pay attention to the signals from my body.

I knew I had to change the way I approached life. Youth can absorb many things, but as you get older and have more responsibilities, your frenetic lifestyle catches up with you. You feel overwhelmed by the years of overextending in all directions and realize that operating at this level is not only unsustainable, but also not much fun.

I owned and managed my own fitness studios in central London at the time and started to notice that I wasn't the only one feeling like this. I saw clients who—no matter how many yoga, Pilates, or other fitness classes they attended—would quickly rebound to feeling stressed and at the edge of burnout.

I began to seek sustainable practices that went more deeply into nervous-system regulation, which influences how you experience life. And I aimed to do so without the tyranny of willpower or enforced positive thinking, which only serve to disconnect you, as they don't allow you to feel the full range of human emotions: love, anger, curiosity, spontaneity, lust, fear, and grief. I studied and researched and then trialed my findings on myself and my clients over the years, and I honed and tweaked my approach to arrive at The Human Method: a radical relearning system that uses a combination of somatic movement, breathwork, and restorative practices to harmonize the mind and body. The method was originally developed to help people with illness or injury-rehab and mobility issues. However, I noticed that there was also a need to help those who were experiencing chronic stress, burnout, anxiety, and trauma. So I created The Soothe Program, which is designed to help people regulate their nervous system and reduce the symptoms of these conditions.

My clients have had powerful results with The Soothe Program, and I want to share my knowledge so that you can feel the benefits too.

What is The Soothe Program?

My practice is rooted in a somatic approach. "Somatic" means relating to the body. Somatic movement uses motion to help people connect with their bodies and their emotions. It can be helpful for those who are dealing with pain, stress, or anxiety.

The word "somatic" comes from the Greek *soma*, which means "body." Somatic movement therapy is based on the idea that the body and mind are not separate, but instead are interconnected. When we experience emotions, they can manifest in our bodies in the form of tension, pain, or other physical symptoms. Somatic movement can help us to release these physical symptoms and reconnect with our bodies in a more mindful way.

In the years since first developing and practicing The Soothe Program to focus on nervous-system regulation I have been able to self-regulate my emotions in a more compassionate way, so that I can deal with stresses as they arise instead of storing habitual patterns in my body, which gave me intense emotions until they became unbearable. I am now more honest in my relationships and able to talk about difficult matters without blowing things apart. I sleep better, I no longer suffer from chronic anxiety and I understand the importance of rest. For the first time in my life, I feel at peace with who I am and where I am. With this knowledge, I smoothly navigated the sale of my fitness studios, which I had been running for thirteen years; hitting menopause; moving my specialist work to an online clinic; the Covid-19 pandemic and moving out of London, where I was born and bought up, a total of fifty-five years, to live by the sea.

This isn't to say that I don't worry about things or am not sad or despondent sometimes. While writing this book there have been far too many deaths of dear ones, illness, sadness, war in Ukraine and the Middle East, humanitarian crises around the world, the ever-growing climate crisis, an energy crisis and a cost-of-living crisis. I have learned to stop my rumination in its tracks, so that I am no longer paralyzed with anxiety about what might come. In my own life and in those of my clients, I have found that allowing your thoughts to go round and round in your head or pushing down your emotions results in mental anguish. It also means that you don't live in an authentic way, embracing all aspects of what makes you who you are. I believe such inauthentic living stops you having meaningful relationships with yourself and others.

I have now learned to tend to myself when intense feelings occur and to metabolize my emotions out of my body. Once I have soothed myself, I am able to make decisions from a much calmer mind. I have learned to enjoy the

process of living, so that I don't wait for that one day when
all the things I want for my life will finally align. I now have
easy in-body or embodied solutions, instead of seeking the
next external fad in the hope that it will soothe me. I am
better able to cultivate a more compassionate relationship
with myself and with my life.

How can The Soothe Program help you?

Instead of looking after ourselves throughout our lives, we
mainly tend to ourselves only when we are broken. We don't
stop to ask, "Why am I feeling anxious, sad, or emotionally
tired?" We don't stop to ask, "Why do we all put up with our
collective lack of ease?" We push through, with our bodies
feeling tense and sore, our brains constantly overstimulated.
We might feel personally grateful for and content with our
own circumstances, but at the same time we may feel hugely
ill at ease with the bombardment of news about the worst of
humanity. It lodges deep within our bodies, and slowly our
ability to feel at peace is chipped away.

I have discovered that much of that sense of unease comes
from our overworked nervous systems. Unprocessed emotions become stuck, causing us to live in a state of constant
high alertness, or hypervigilance. You might feel extremely
sensitive to your surroundings and yet push your feelings
down, because you have been taught to ignore unpleasant
sensations. Or you feel so confused by the conflicting messages out there that you don't trust your feelings. You can't
afford to feel overwhelmed, for there is never enough time to
tend to yourself, so you simply say, "I can't think about that
right now" or "I'll deal with this at the end of the day," and

you get on with it. You hope that sleep will reboot your tired mind, but there is so much to process at the end of the day that you can't quite settle into peaceful slumber. For some people, alertness turns into apathy and an increasing lack of enthusiasm, with the spark no longer burning bright.

Soothe will teach you how to listen to your body's signals so that you will be able to metabolize your emotions and live with more energy, enthusiasm, and joy. Our dominant culture teaches us that *the mind rules the body*, and while I understood this conceptually, I now embody this understanding. Everything you think is dictated by what you feel and by your life experiences. I don't believe it is possible to *think* yourself out of a *feeling* state. You can contextualize and rationalize whatever has happened to you, but to change behavior in the long term you need to engage your mind and body or, as I prefer to call it, your "whole self."

Using the somatic principles of The Soothe Program, I will walk you through how your body and mind work together, provide lessons to help you connect the two and introduce you to micro-practices to incorporate into your day. You will learn to *soothe* with your body, body sensing, the breath, touch, movement, rest, nourishment, and connection; the first part of the book will give you the knowledge to fully understand your nervous system and its needs.

Once you know the *what*, the *how*, and the *why*, you will have the ability to cultivate new experiences that will soothe your nervous system. You will be able to let go of habits that you no longer need and, using the daily lessons in the second part of the book, be able to move through life processing stresses as they come, to avoid storing them in your body; and you will live with awareness and an integrated body and mind. The case studies included in *Soothe* will help to demonstrate how this method has worked for my clients, and will show how it can be applied to anyone. In the interest of preserving privacy, all identities have been anonymized, but I hope you'll be able to see yourself in some of the case studies and know that you can find a way to healing and balance, too.

Soothe goes back to the basics of how to be human. You perceive yourself and the world around you through your whole body's responses. Your body is continually negotiating its relationship to gravity, always in motion, as you subconsciously try to find your balance and equilibrium. The whole body is a web of interconnections and rhythms, from the electrical frequency of brain waves to the flow of blood, the pulsing of cells, the chemical responses of hormones, the release of synovial fluid in the joints and the slow movement of lymph as it carries waste out of the body. Moving the body, and tending to it on a regular basis, will enable you to function in an optimum way. And as you embark on a new chapter of normality where you are more conscious of your health and well-being than ever before, what could be a more exciting prospect than that?

Time and again, I see how teaching people to soothe themselves transforms lives. Now I want to help readers understand why learning to self-soothe will be the most empowering practice you will encounter.

Let us begin.

Part 1

Soothe

1

Your Body

We've moved from wisdom to knowledge, and now
we're moving from knowledge to information,
and that information is so partial—that we're
creating incomplete human beings.

Vandana Shiva, Indian activist[1]

Many years ago, before I taught clients, I used to practice hot
yoga. Once, in a ninety-minute class, I experienced a transfor-
mative moment, but not in the way people usually associate
with yoga. We were about halfway through the class, about
to start the standing-pose section. I was tired, because being
in a hot room for so long *is* tiring: that challenge is precisely
why hot yoga appeals to its audience, including me at that
time. This form of yoga is a test of endurance, which chimes
well with the work-hard city-living culture. At the time I was
in a job that was well paid but gave me no purpose. I would
turn up for work each day but felt that I produced nothing
of value. My marriage had run its course and I had to insti-
gate a difficult conversation about going our separate ways. I
didn't like to be still, because it forced me to think about the
direction of my life and that caused me too much anxiety. So

here I was, in a hot-yoga class, trying to distract myself from my ongoing mental turmoil.

The instructions were centered on doing more of everything: stretch more, lock out your joints, expand more, actively contract a muscle and breathe more fully. The instructor told us to move into tree. She gave us step-by-step instructions: stand on one leg, pick the other leg up, bend at the knee, and press the foot into the side of the standing leg. Push your bent knee out. It looks as if your standing leg is a tree trunk; this leg supports your weight. Then pull up your quads. "Now," she said, "bend the supporting leg and bring your fingertips to the floor." I was unconvinced of this, but my inner dialogue was saying, "It's okay. She is the teacher; she is trained in yoga and anatomy. She knows what I am capable of, because she is certified."

I came up onto the ball of my foot on my standing leg, as instructed; a small part of my foot supported my entire weight. I bent this knee and started to crouch down. I realized there had been no mention of my other knee—the one bent and externally rotated out from the hip. What did I do with it? Pushing was the last instruction, so I did that. I finally breathed when I almost fell to the ground and my fingers touched down. Somehow I did it; the ordeal was over. But the teacher was standing next to me. "Now come up, the same way you went down," she said.

I didn't know how to do this, but I attempted to, because the teacher had told me to do so. I started to unbend the supporting leg. I came back up on the ball of the foot—every part of me was telling me not to do this; the other knee was pressed out and my pelvis felt like it was splitting apart. Then my knee let out an audible ripping sound, as if I had torn something underneath the kneecap. I let out a silent shriek; after all, I didn't want to embarrass myself in class. I put both feet on the ground and looked at my teacher. I was cross at her, and I was cross at myself. She could see that I was angry and started to walk backward, away from me. I hobbled out of the class, feeling like a yoga failure, but I was also confused as to why I had let a stranger convince me to practice something that I sensed was not going to turn out well. Why did I relinquish my own responsibility for my body to someone else?

This scenario is not particular to yoga; but in this class and in many other fitness activities that I used to take part in, I would check out of my mind and relinquish responsibility for my body to the teacher. In that particular case, I ignored the warning signals that my knee was sending me. I ignored the sensations in my ankle, which was unable to find its balance; the tension in my calf and thigh muscles— signs that my body was telling my brain this felt unsafe, and that they were bracing to mitigate the imminent damage. I was also ignoring the fact that I was holding my breath and feeling anxious, because I had exercised little skill in coming down to the floor. I wasn't going to be able to replicate this movement because I had no sensory-motor understanding of how I got here, so I didn't know how to come back up again. I felt under pressure because of the class's fast pace, and because my imagination convinced me that everyone was watching me. There was no time for me to figure all of this out. I did not practice with attention, but instead forced myself, even though my internal alarm bells were going wild.

Here's the problem with this approach: our thinking is

based on the experiences that have shaped us. My experiences at that time were that I was a speed freak: I worked long hours, sitting at a computer for most of the day, eyes glued to the screen, with the back of my neck sore, my shoulders hunched up to my ears and my head positioned forward of my spine. As I've said, I didn't love my job, but I put in extra effort to prove that I was eager and indispensable. I would go out almost every night to unwind from a day job that gave me no purpose. I regularly went to bed past midnight, and I drank a lot of coffee to keep me awake throughout the day. I forgot to eat, then would overeat in one sitting because I was famished. I drank more alcohol than I meant to and took recreational drugs (don't judge me, it was the 1990s) to help me dampen down my noisy head, because I could not bear the sadness of the world, the weight of my own sorrow and the feeling that I was wasting my life, living with no purpose. Most of the time I was stressed or anxious, and my exercise had an element of punishment about it. It was almost as if I wanted to beat the anxiety and sadness out of my body.

Back to the hot-yoga room: in hindsight, thinking "I can push through this" was not an adequate strategy to stop me injuring myself. Paying attention to the communication between my body and my nervous system would have given me the necessary information to make better choices.

In this one yoga class I came face-to-face with the many ideas that I had about myself—ideas that I had formed over a lifetime:

- I should not trust the signals coming from my body, because they were primal.

- My mind should override signals from my body because my mind was more sophisticated than my body.
- My body must be forced to achieve an outcome, at all costs.
- I was wrong for not being agile.
- I was rubbish at everything.
- I should obey my teacher because she had more knowledge than I did.
- I didn't want to look foolish in front of other people.
- I didn't want to have a confrontation in a public class, with a teacher who meant well.
- I still felt stressed and anxious.

A yoga class that I thought would teach me to reduce my stress levels instead tripped me into a vortex of negative thoughts that made me sharply confront many beliefs I held about myself: opinions are formed by my experiences in the world, and these beliefs determine my actions and behavior—signals from my body, be damned!

So how did being unable to come up from a yoga pose take me down this black hole? Our attitudes to our minds and bodies so often treat them as two entirely separate entities, and we feel we must prioritize one over the other. The harmony between the two is often unknown to us, and this leads to dissociation and feeling ill at ease in the world. We find no refuge in ourselves, either in mind or in body, and therefore we have nowhere to call home. Movement is fundamental to who we are as human beings, because how we move is all about how we move through life. The class didn't help me to address the reasons for my stress and anxiety; it

just displaced one action for another type of action, all in
the service of keeping me busy.

We live in a culture where doing too much is encouraged:
too much work, too much socializing, too many different
activities, too much food, too much alcohol . . . and no time
to process any of it. All in service of seeming to *live* more.
Because our senses are so heightened with stimuli, we only
seem to have two speeds: full throttle or exhausted. And
both speeds are socially approved states. How many people
do you know who push their bodies to the max with work,
and then again in their nonwork lives, because being productive or busy is seen as the most valid way to spend our
time?

Sometimes it seems that our physical practices support
this culture, too: there is meditation to make employees
more productive, spinning classes with a spiritual happy
ending, yoga to sell yoga-wear, and other spiritual knick-
knacks, in an attempt to give our lives meaning.

But what if ambition, speed, and acquisition were not the
only human goals? What if we also valued sensing, exploring, learning, the beauty of the process, resting, creating,
pausing, resetting, repairing, calibrating, or even compas-
sionately *being*?

Back then, no matter what activity I did or how much I
practiced it, I was still stressed and anxious. Yoga, running,
and boxing made me feel exhilarated for a while, but soon I
was back to the habits I had formed over the years, in order
to enable me to function in my surrounding environment.
This was why I was feeling stressed and anxious. I had
conditioned myself to expect a physical class several times
a week to transform my mind and body, but what I really

needed to do was examine my approach to life—and what influenced that approach.

The experience in the hot-yoga class awakened in me a desire to find out how I could transform myself without having to adopt yet another "self-improvement" regime. I had tried so many different regimes, and while I would typically manage to stick with one for a month or even a year, I kept reverting to my stressed and anxious habits because I was familiar with them. Each new regime would demand more effort, because my mind had to push my body. Then my body would rebel, and the cycle would repeat.

My seeking led me to learn more about the nervous system and how it works. I immersed myself in *embodied*, or *somatic*, movement and *interoception*. The latter is the sensory system that provides information about the internal condition of the body.

I found that modern living tends to overlook interoception—I certainly had done, until that fateful day in the yoga class. We are more likely to be aware of *exteroception*, which provides information about the external body, such as your environment and temperature; and of *proprioception* (the best known of the three terms), which provides information about the body's force, pressure and location in space. This allows you balance, coordination, and agility, so that you can move your limbs without looking at them.

Interoception, which is focused on internal feeling, is the missing ingredient that can enable you to feel wholly engaged and curious about how you do what you do. Without tapping into your interoceptive sense, you end up using your mind to force your body to push through, regardless of the fallout it causes. I often see clients who have a tendency to separate their physical sensations from their internal experiences. This is a familiar way of being, in our fast-paced world, but it can also be a barrier to feeling truly connected to ourselves and our bodies.

The idea of the separate body and mind

Where does this separation of the mind and body come from? There are many possible factors. We live in a culture that values the mind over the body. This can lead us to believe that our thoughts and emotions are more important than our physical sensations. If we have experienced trauma, we may have learned to dissociate from our bodies as a way of coping with the painful memories. If we experience chronic pain, we may learn to ignore our physical sensations as a way of handling the discomfort.

The philosophical concept of the split between body and mind originated with the French philosopher René Descartes (1596–1650), who argued that the mind and body are two separate substances, with the mind being immaterial and the body being material.[2] This separation of the mind and body can have a profound impact on our lives. It can lead to us feeling disconnected from ourselves, from our bodies and from the world around us. It can also make it difficult to manage pain, stress, and anxiety.

When I refer to the "mind," I am using the modern definition by neuroscientist Dr. Susan Greenfield, who describes it as "the personalization of the brain through its unique dynamic configuration of your neural connections that are, in turn, driven by your unique experiences."[3] In simple terms, the neural pathways of your brain are uniquely shaped by the life you have lived. Your idea of reality is based on your life experiences.

An example of this might be that you were brought up to be fearful of dogs. To you, dogs represent fear. You might have read or heard stories to reinforce your fear—for instance, a news story about a dog biting a child—or had a particularly savage neighborhood dog that barked through the fence every time you walked past. Perhaps the culture you were brought up in deemed dogs to be dirty and feral, and believed that their savage nature had to be strictly controlled. Now, when you see a dog, you conjure up all this information that you have about them. Your body also reacts to this information: you will *feel* this fear of dogs in your body, even before you have had time to *think* about your response. Your heart races, your hands feel sweaty and you want to run away every time you see a dog, because your brain draws in response on the ideas that you have about all dogs. Your hands clench into fists, your throat gets tight and your breathing becomes shallow. These bodily signals inform your brain that you are in danger. This is an integrated view of the mind and body, which draws on all your experiences to allow a fast body response to get you out of danger.

In the above scenario I am describing myself. I was terrified of dogs, but over the years my friends acquired dogs and I became better acquainted with them around the home and saw how loving, trusting, and vulnerable they are. I encountered the cutest Boston terrier puppy, who was soft and friendly. I was totally smitten—so much so that this adorable encounter sowed the seeds for me now owning three Boston terriers, who enjoy an elevated status in my household. I replaced my fearful experiences of dogs with new, more pleasurable experiences of being around them. This enabled me to change my ideas *about* dogs. Now, instead of being fearful, I am thrilled to be around them.

What this means is that your responses are based on your bodily sensations and your past experiences. Rather than your *mind* thinking about what to do and then informing your body, your body sends signals upward. Assuming that you are not in danger, what I encourage you to do is pause and consider what your bodily signals actually mean. Going back to the dog scenario, I saw a small and vulnerable puppy with its big eyes and needy vulnerability, and my body softened and I smiled. This signaled that there was no danger from this instance of "dog." When you can attune to your bodily responses and become curious about them, you can change your emotions and your thoughts and meet life in the moment.

We have the legacy of a mechanistic view of our *bodies* as separate entities from our *minds*. This separation of mind and body also has its roots in the study of human anatomy by dissection, originating in the eighteenth century. The scientific mapping of the body—such as identifying specific muscles connected to either end of a specific bone, or examining the gut purely for its function as an organ of digestion—is useful to visualize the different parts of the body. But this process has inadvertently encouraged us to view our bodies purely as machines of flesh and bone, ignoring the complete human condition. Many of us are confused or unaware of how our bodies *feel*, because the mind is given top billing and is always thought to have more awareness and insight than the body. This mechanistic outlook ignores interoception—the process by which our brain interprets signals from the body's internal organs, muscles, and tissues. These signals are then used to create a representation of the body's state, which can be used to inform our thoughts, feelings, and actions.

The mechanistic view of the "body" doesn't shed light on how the mind, nervous system, organs, and muscles interact, and on the ongoing communication between all the bodily systems that make up the self, which includes body and mind. That we are a brain with a body is still the prevalent paradigm, although we now understand that we are more a body with a brain. Moving away from the mechanistic view of your body is an important step in understanding how to care deeply for yourself.

Breath practice with mechanistic cueing

Try this breath practice as a step-by-step physical exercise:

1 Before you start, check in with how you are feeling now.
2 Come to sit or lie down. Let your eyes close.
3 Inhale through your nose for four counts and push your belly out.
4 Exhale through your nose for four counts by pulling your belly in.
5 Do this three times.
6 Now slowly open your eyes. How do you feel? A bit out of breath? Can you feel the effort you made through your belly muscles? Do you feel peaceful? Probably not.

Somatic breath practice

Now try this practice by paying attention to your bodily or interoceptive sensations:

1   Either lie on the floor or come up to sit, letting your eyes close. Bring your attention to your breathing as the air passes in and out through your nostrils.

2   Inhale gradually through the nose for a slow count of four—as you do so, let your belly rise.

3   Exhale gradually through the nose for a slow count of four and let your belly fall.

4   Continue with this pace of breathing but, as you practice, think about the pulsating movement of a jellyfish; make each breath softer, and imagine that your lungs are expanding into the ribs on the inhale and retracting back from the ribs on the exhale.

5   Do this a few times until you are ready to open your eyes. How do you feel now?

The first practice feels like you are performing it with your external body, with the habits that you have accumulated over the years. This version takes considerable effort and doesn't feel particularly pleasant. The result is that you probably still feel the same—there was no shift in your mental state.

The second practice feels softer and cultivates awareness of your internal body, with less muscular or external body effort. The chances are that you feel calmer and more connected afterward.

Embracing interoception

As we have seen, interoception is the perception of the state of our internal body and it significantly influences many areas of our lives, such as self-regulation, mental health and social connection.

Our self-image—or the idea we have of ourselves—is made up of awareness of our physical body, feeling, senses, movement, and thought.[4] When we listen to our internal signals, we have a better chance of achieving a nuanced awareness that enables us to discern, to differentiate, to be in a state of curiosity, explore creativity, and embrace novelty. We can better interpret our feelings and make well-informed decisions in any situation. When we ignore these signals and push through regardless, there is no expansion of our ideas; we stay stuck in our beliefs about ourselves, which continue to have a limiting effect on our experience.

The traditional idea of a brain controlling a body to do its bidding is incorrect. In my experience, a more useful idea is to think about your body in a continual conversation with your brain, which is more accurate. The brain's job is to keep us alive by budgeting our resources.[5] It does this by receiving data-streams from the body, giving real-time information about how we are at any given time. This continual two-way dialogue allows the brain to adjust your levels of resources, such as glucose and water, to keep you functioning optimally in an ever-changing environment.

Your brain is constantly predicting what will happen to you next; it does this to maintain the stability of your body's internal environment, even when the external environment changes. Interoception—or your brain's representation of the sensations arising from your body—is the sensory result of the brain's attempts to regulate your body's internal systems. It is central to everything, from thought to emotions to decision-making and our sense of self.

You feel what your brain believes[6]

The neuroscientist David Marr first proposed in the 1970s the idea that our brains predict. Marr argued that the brain constantly tries to make sense of the world by predicting what will happen next. This idea was popularized by the neuroscientist Lisa Feldman Barrett,[7] and her research is hugely important to my approach and will give you an understanding of how and why *Soothe* is so effective in changing your habits.

Your brain doesn't simply react to the world around you. It is constantly trying to anticipate what is going to happen, so that it can keep your budget of resources in balance. Your body sends signals to your brain that you do not consciously notice. These signals tell your brain about your internal state, such as your heart rate, blood pressure, and body temperature.

In the nineteenth century scientists believed that the brain was a passive organ responding to environmental stimuli. This view of the brain as reactive to situations was supported by the observation that the brain's neurons fire in response to sensory input. However, in the early twentieth century scientists realized that the brain is not simply a passive organ. They discovered that the brain is constantly active, even when we are not experiencing any external stimuli. This activity is the brain's way of generating predictions about the world.

As your brain sits in your skull with no access to the outside world, it creates maps of your body from the sense data coming in, and from your prior experiences. It predicts what is happening and uses your sense data to confirm or refine it. This model helps your brain predict what will happen next so that it can take steps to keep you safe and healthy.

Imagine this scenario: you are in your garden and want to move a big, heavy, dark-gray pot to the other side of the path. This pot is similar in color, size, and shape to all the other pots in your garden. You have moved them around before and understand how heavy they are. You bend down and physically prepare to pick up the heavy pot. Still, as soon as your fingers connect to the pot, before you even attempt to pick it up, you become aware that it is made of plastic, which means it is much lighter than the ceramic pots with a similar appearance. Your senses and your brain's prediction are not in alignment; you have already started to move; you lift this pot with more force than you need and have to steady yourself. If you were moving more slowly and allowing all inputs to process, you might be able to adjust the effort that you use as you pick up the pot.

Your brain issues predictions of the weight of the pot, based on your prior experience of the different pots in your garden. Your sensory input informs your brain that this pot is much lighter and requires less effort to lift it off the floor. Now your brain must update its understanding of this lighter pot, and remap it in your brain's model of your body in the world. The next time you go to pick up a pot, you might tap it with your foot to see what it is made of, or visually recognize the lighter material it is created from.

Brain predictions and sensory input are in a dance of influencing and refining each other. Our brains are constantly making predictions about the world around us. These predictions include our own body's movements. If our brains were merely reactive, they would have to wait for sensory input from our bodies before issuing motor commands to muscles. This would be slow and inefficient. By giving motor predictions, our brains can anticipate the need to move and issue motor commands more quickly.

This ability to issue motor predictions is essential for our survival. For example, if we see a snake, our brain can give motor predictions to move out of the way before we can consciously think about it. This fast action enables us to react to threats quickly and effectively.

The interoceptive networks in your brain, when explained very simply, are a coming together of body-budget regions and the primary interoceptive cortex, which deals with sensory inputs, working to keep you alive. You use some of your energy resources every time you move externally or even internally. You don't have to physically move to use your resources. If, for example, someone you know is judgmental of your choices, the next time they walk toward you, your brain predicts that you need energy and releases cortisol that floods your bloodstream with glucose, so that your muscles lengthen and contract to allow you to run away from the perceived unpleasantness. Even the thought of someone saying something judgmental can potentially use up your body's budget of resources.

The people around you can also regulate your body's budget in a positive way. When you spend time with your partner, you start to synchronize your breathing and heartbeat with theirs, reducing the activation of your body-budget regions. Everything you do, think about, imagine, see, hear, touch, and smell, and every person you interact with, has budgetary consequences for your body. These external and internal elements inform your brain about the world and help to shape it.

You replenish your budget by eating well, drinking enough liquid to hydrate, and sleeping. You also reduce your body-budget "spend" by passing time with loved ones and doing something enjoyable. Understanding this integrated brain-and-body state is invaluable.

What is the consequence of living with the prevalent view of a separation between body and mind? Since I began teaching, my clients have shown me—through the tension in their muscles, jaw, and shoulders, the knots in their stomachs and their inability to breathe to their total capacity—that the physical body marks the events and habits that make up our lives. Our bodies are shaped by how we feel, what we eat, how we rest, our behaviors, our habits and our environment. A cultivated interoceptive sense has wide-ranging repercussions for our well-being. Recent studies suggest that listening to signals from our internal organs allows us to self-regulate our emotions and keep depression and anxiety at bay.[8]

Interoception is a complex process; it is the bridge between the mind and the body and is essential for survival. Willpower or rationalization using your cognitive mind alone cannot change your physical or mental state in the long term; you must involve all of you—and that includes listening to your bodily signals.

Your brain maps your body

Your brain maps your body through a process called somato-topy. This is the organization of the body's sensory and motor information in the brain.

The somatosensory cortex is the part of the brain that receives sensory information from the body. It is located just behind the forehead in the parietal lobe. The somatosensory cortex is divided into a map of the body, with each part of the body being represented by a specific area of the cortex.

The motor cortex is the part of the brain that controls movement. It is located in the frontal lobe, just in front of the somatosensory cortex. It is also divided into a map of the body, with each part of the body being represented by a specific area of the cortex.

The somatotopy of the brain is elastic. It can change over time, based on our experiences. For example, if we lose a limb, the brain can reorganize the somatosensory cortex to map the remaining parts of the body onto the area that was previously dedicated to the missing limb.

The somatotopy of the brain is also influenced by our emotions. For example, when we experience pain, the soma-tosensory cortex becomes more active. This is because the brain is paying more attention to the painful area of the body. Interestingly your body cannot feel exactly where it ends. The area around your body that you can feel is called the peripersonal space. It is a bubble of space that surrounds your body and is defined by your senses.

Your senses—such as touch, proprioception and vision—work together to create your peripersonal space. Touch tells you about the contact between your body and the outside world. Proprioception tells you about the position and movement of your body parts. Vision tells you about the objects in your environment.

The peripersonal space is not fixed. It can change depending on your attention, your emotions and your environment. If you are wearing a hat, you somehow know how much to duck under a door in order not to knock it off—your peripersonal space has expanded to include that object. If you are in a dangerous situation, your peripersonal space may shrink to protect you.

Your body likes to have feedback from the floor and walls to soothe the nervous system, because it provides a sense of security and grounding. When you are feeling stressed or anxious, your body goes into a state of hyper-arousal. This means that your heart rate and breathing increase, your muscles tense up and your senses become heightened. This is a normal reaction to danger, but it can feel unpleasant and make it difficult to think clearly. Feedback from the floor and walls can help to calm the nervous system by providing a sense of stability and support. When we feel our bodies pressed against a solid surface, it sends a message to our brains that we are safe and secure. This can help to slow down our heart rate and breathing, relax our muscles and reduce our anxiety.

Case study: Savannah

I first met Savannah when she came to my studios in central London for one-to-one sessions. She worked in banking and had reached the point of burnout, a condition that involves increased anxiety levels, erratic sleep patterns, and tiredness. She had started

a new job with significantly more responsibilities. She was working across global time zones, switching on her laptop early in the
morning and still checking in to work twelve hours later. Her sleep
was squeezed, and work was always on her mind.

Savannah recognized that feeling on the edge of burnout
wasn't healthy or sustainable. She often felt overwhelmed, anxious,
and even a little lost; this manifested in her moving physically into
a protected state, where her shoulders were rounded and she collapsed into her front body. This, in turn, affected her breathing,
which became shallower. Like many of my clients, to "fix" herself
and sleep better Savannah would throw herself into extreme fitness, spinning, and HIIT classes, which left her aching and exhausted
the next day. She hoped that intensely physical classes would ex-
haust her into sleep, but when her head hit the pillow she was
thinking about the financial markets, the dollar against the pound,
and what she had to do first thing in the morning.

Her job was to find solutions, so she approached her life
similarly by being the strong one who could organize things for
everyone else. Her wish was to adopt a healthier attitude, but
every time she tried, work would intrude, and she had no energy to
continue her good habits. She would feel bad about herself, which
further increased her desire to excel on all fronts, to *work* herself
into a better person.

Savannah was so accustomed to using her clever mind to
solve problems and organize others that she had forgotten how
to tend to herself. We embarked on a series of private sessions,
so that I could look at her breathing patterns and she would be
able to gently notice how she moved and where she held tension.
When you send your focused attention to your physical body, you
are perceiving what is being sensed, which in turn changes your
sensations. In this instance it was to accommodate her breath. I

showed Savannah how she could incorporate simple strategies into her day to soothe her mind and body from the intensity of her working life. The more she could let go of the effects of the stressors throughout the day, the more she could let go of her working day in the evening and regain her ability to sleep. Savannah and I were working together as the pandemic hit, and we kept going through the ensuing lockdowns, as I was able to teach her online.

Her commitment to consistent deep care meant that when she lost both of her parents just as we were coming out of the pandemic—and remember that we were discouraged from gatherings and care-home visits—her practice with me enabled her to navigate the trauma and loss, with compassion for herself. She became someone who could look after herself, perform well in her demanding job and create healthy boundaries around her work and personal life. She cultivated resilience and was better able to metabolize her emotions through her body, rather than shutting them down.

Savannah now feels content, light of body, spirit, and mind. She continues to attend my online classes and she books into every retreat because she understands that tending to yourself isn't a short-term hack; deep care is a lifelong process that will help you live to your full potential. Most of us choose to emphasize a particular aspect of ourselves. It is usually the shiny front end, which shows that we are in control and leading a life full of external experiences: travel, shopping, and going out to fancy restaurants. We try to push down anything that doesn't fit the idea of the person we want to project to the world. However, when you embrace all aspects of who you are—including the less shiny parts of yourself—and become more curious about these parts, you can stop this internal war between the different parts of you and are better able to cultivate a more compassionate relationship with yourself.

Being in a compassionate relationship with yourself enables you to be in a compassionate and authentic relationship with others, and with your environment. This means that you are not in a battle to be an idealized version of yourself, but are accepting of the more real, human version. Doesn't this sound a more peaceful way to live?

When you are rested, you can use your resources to direct your attention in a focused manner. But when you are exhausted, you tend to default to the habitual strategies that have kept you functioning in your environment. Learning how to do things differently takes effort, and when you are wired and tired you have no energy to query or change.

Your nervous system

We'll look at "rest" in Chapter 6 of this book, but for now let's learn how to "listen in" by looking at the human body through an embodied or integrated focus.

While learning the Latin names for muscles is useful, we must go underneath the layer of terminology to get a sense of the interwoven relationship of your body and gain a deeper understanding of the dynamic, complex, multidimensional, interconnected, and deeply profound organism you are.

How will understanding your body as an organism help, when you simply want to learn about how to soothe your nervous system and live better right now? Well, without understanding the interconnectedness of all your body's systems from the moment of your conception, you will forever be in a push-pull relationship with your mind and your body. And it is this battle that is exhausting and exasperating you.

So let's dive in.

This interrelational organization of a human being starts from conception. It develops in the embryo and continues throughout an entire life. An important part of my work is educating clients about their body and how it interacts with their mind—and that means understanding themselves as an integrated system, with all parts working collaboratively. I teach people with nervous-system regulation issues, whose symptoms might be chronic anxiety, stress, or sleep problems. They might be managing pain or attempting to move on from deeply held traumatic events in their lives. I will be referring to the *nervous system* many times, so let's define exactly what I mean by this.

Your nervous system includes your brain, your spinal cord and all the connections to your organs and body, and from the organs and body back to your brain and spinal cord. Your nervous system is a continuous loop of communication. It was once thought that we are a brain driving a body, but it turns out that we have more information coming up from the body to the brain, or a *bottom-up* approach, than we do from the brain to the body, known as a *top-down* approach.[9]

Your nervous system is traditionally described in two parts: the *central nervous system*, which is your brain and spinal cord; and the *peripheral nervous system*, which refers to the nerves that extend to your body. Your peripheral nervous system branches into the *somatic nervous system* and *the autonomic nervous system*.

The somatic nervous system relates to the muscles that you can control, the nerves throughout your body that carry information from your senses, including sound and touch. The autonomic nervous system is the part of your nervous system that connects your brain to your internal organs. It has three further branches, which are:

- *Sympathetic nervous system*: sometimes called the stress response, which I find an emotive term. I prefer to think of this as either your arousal system or the "go" part of your nervous system. It activates body processes that prepare you for action. This system is responsible for your body's "fight, freeze, or flight" response.

- *Parasympathetic nervous system*: this part of your autonomic nervous system is responsible for the "rest, repair, and digest" body processes. It is the brake system that counters the arousal system. I prefer to think of this as the "recover" or "no-go" part of your system.

- *Enteric nervous system*: this is a network of neurons that line the gut and is a complex system that isn't fully understood. It is sometimes called the second brain because it can function outside the central nervous system. This part of your nervous system is responsible for digestion, absorption, and immunity and plays an important role in mood regulation, as it is connected to the brain's emotional centers.

Your nervous system regulates, and is influenced by, all other biological systems of your body. If this array of seemingly disparate parts of the nervous system is a bit confusing, don't worry!

The key takeaway is that your nervous system and your body are in a continuous interconnected communication loop—and if you want to experience sustainable change, look to the nervous system and the communication from your body to it, and from your nervous system back to your body. This continuous connection is there in the embryonic development of a human being, which helps us to understand the interwoven, multilayered way in which we function. Let's look at this next.

How your body is formed

After a sperm fertilizes an egg, the cells divide and form a two-disc layer inside two fluid-filled cavities. A third layer then develops in the midline, creating a front, middle, and back of the body:

- The front layer is called the endoderm. It gives rise to the digestive and respiratory systems, the liver, the pancreas and the inner lungs.
- The middle layer is called the mesoderm. It gives rise to the circulatory, skeletal, muscular, cardiovascular, and reproductive systems. It also differentiates into connective tissue.
- The back layer is called the ectoderm. It gives rise to the nervous system and the skin.

Each layer has distinctive qualities. The endoderm is involved in nutrition, absorption, and secretion. The ectoderm can sense, communicate, react, and make choices. The mesoderm holds the body together and allows movement. It is the action body, offering support, and the ability to move dynamically toward food and away from danger.

An important takeaway from this is that these three layers all originate from the same tissue. They develop different functions, but they are all interconnected throughout your life. To me, this shows how complex and interwoven the human body is, from development onward.

The first system to develop in the embryo is the circulatory system. This makes sense, because the circulatory system is responsible for getting nutrients to the cells and removing waste. The embryo forms by folding and rolling into itself—the external becomes internal, and the internal becomes external, there is no separation between the two—which creates cavities and tubes that enable different organ systems to evolve.

The human fetus is suspended in fluid and attached to its mother by the umbilical cord at its navel. The fetus takes in nourishment and rids itself of waste through this connection.

From the center of the fetus, the neck develops and travels both upward to the head and downward to what will become the tailbone; the upper limbs develop and then the lower limbs. Through movement, the fetus's nervous system develops to help organize the functions taking place in the embryo. The first nerves of the body are the vestibular nerves of the inner ear, which register the environment by balance and spatial orientation. The sensory information is processed in the nervous system. The motor nerves develop before the sensory nerves. The feedback of movement is essential for future development of the human baby: physical, sensory, perceptual, psychological, and mental.

Movement comes first, then the sensory feedback about that movement. Movement is the original awareness.[10] The fetus detects the movements of the mother and is moved by the mother, which, in turn, influences the movement of the fetus. The sensory nerves from the body to the brain signal the motor nerves to contract and release muscle. This communication through the nervous system is how the fetus defines its identity as separate from its mother. Movement is detected in every body cell—in the bones, joints, muscles, and connective tissue—and through interoceptive nerves in the organs.

This relationship of the fetus with its environment gives us an idea of the whole body thinking, sensing, and moving, to understand where it is in relationship to gravity, space, time, and energy. Having a sense of how we arrived here, through our development, can help to relate to the forces that organized our systems and continue to do so throughout our lives.

Another important system that is fundamental to understanding the human body as an interconnected system is the *fascial system*. Fascia falls under the umbrella term of *connective tissue*, along with ligaments, tendons, cartilage, bone, and blood. Connective tissues are those that bind, support and connect other tissues and organs in the body. Fascia is a network of wet connective tissue that sits immediately under the skin, webbing the entire body and giving us our shape and structure. It wraps around the bones, cartilage, organs, and muscles, but also travels right through them. A visual metaphor might be to think of sashimi rolled in a stretchy, juicy plastic wrap that can move in all directions. The plastic wrap covers the surface of the sashimi but is also entwined through it. Think of it as gliding, sliding structures within other gliding and sliding structures.

Fascia is a band of connective tissue beneath the skin that attaches, stabilizes, encloses, and separates muscles and other internal organs. It is one continuous structure that runs through our entire body, from head to toe, without interruption. Trains of fascial lines connect you from the soles of your feet to the crown of your head, and there are also lines that travel laterally and diagonally. The fascial system is rich in sensory nerve endings that detect changes from force, movement, and pressure and send this information to the rest of the body and the brain. The whole body is moving and sensing itself, emphasizing that there is no separation: you are an interconnected organism of component parts that relate one to another, as well as to the whole. When you understand this, you will have a better understanding of how movement and touch are integral to being human. Touch is not just skin-deep; it affects your whole system and is useful in self-care as well as in touch therapies. We will look at this further in Chapter 4.

Fascia is not merely a passive structure; it is also an active one that helps to transmit force and information throughout the body. The fascial system is constantly in motion, even when we are at rest.

I would like to share one further idea with you, to help you move away from a mechanistic view of your body. *Tensegrity* is a structural principle in which a system is held in equilibrium by a network of interconnected tensioned elements. This principle can be applied to the human body. The bones of the body are held in place by the tension of the muscles and fascia. The bones are not rigidly connected to each other, but rather are suspended in a web of soft tissue. This enables the body to move and flex without the bones collapsing.

The spine is a tensegrity structure. The vertebrae are held in place by the tension of the ligaments and muscles. This allows the spine to be flexible and absorb shock. The body's overall shape is determined by the balance of tension in the soft tissues. When the body is in good alignment, the tension in the soft tissues is balanced. This creates a sense of ease and lightness in the body.

The tensegrity principle is a reminder that our bodies are not simply machines. They are complex systems that are held in balance by a network of interconnected elements. When we understand this principle, we can appreciate the beauty and sophistication of our bodies.

Restorative rocking lesson

This chapter has presented you with a lot of information, but in fact the very practice of "listening in" is experiential. Let the information flow through you with a practical lesson. I use this whole-body connection daily and teach it to my clients as an easy way of accessing sensations from their bodies. In technical jargon, you are oscillating through your bones, but I like to call it "jiggling." It was my go-to practice throughout the pandemic when my meditation practice went out of the window—my mind was too fragmented and was of no use in helping me to overcome the locking of my body in fear, which showed up as tense muscle. I still use this practice between my client sessions to help me let go of their emotional load. I also use it at the beginning of a movement practice to help me transition from "go" to "no-go" (see page 34), and before I go to sleep to soften the tensions of my day.

How does it work? Rocking your body can help to release tension and calm an overstimulated nervous system. This is because rocking provides deep pressure and joint compression, which can help to modulate arousal levels, promoting a more balanced and calm state. Rocking engages the "no-go" part of your nervous system, which is the "calming" branch. This is the opposite to the "go" part of your nervous system, which is activated by stress and can lead to increased muscle tension, heart rate, and breathing. When you're tense and tight from trying to contain your feelings, the gentle movement from rocking releases a cascade of endorphins that shifts you into a calming, more relaxed state and lessens the effect of the stressful event. Rocking also increases circulation by sending more oxygen to your joints, which reduces inflammation and pain. And all you need is five to ten minutes to release tension.

Let's just feel this the first time round, and then you can keep trying it so that you make it softer each time. We will come back to this lesson many times in the book, and each time we will add an additional layer of understanding around the movement.

1   Lie on a soft surface—either on a carpeted floor or on a throw on the floor to cushion your spine. Let your legs lengthen out, and let your arms be by your torso, without touching your sides.

2   Notice how you lie on the floor: where on the back of your head do you lie? Are you on the immediate

back of your head or a little more on the left or right
side? Where does your nose point to?

3 Now take your awareness down into your neck and
notice the curve inward. Notice as your neck flows
into the upper spine between your shoulder blades.
Sense into your right shoulder blade: how does this
sit on the floor? Now your left shoulder blade: does
it meet the floor in a different way?

4 Feel how your spine travels through your ribs,
through the upper and mid-back. Now take your
awareness into the lumbar spine or lower back.

5 Allow your awareness to travel into your pelvis:
how does the right side of your pelvis meet the floor
compared to the left side?

6 Take a snapshot of this experience, exactly as it is.

7 Gently press your heels into the ground until your
knees bend a little and your calves come away from
the floor, along with your thighs. Keeping them off the
ground, start to rock your heels on the floor so that the
rocking travels all the way to the back of your head.

8 Pick up the pace to find an easy rocking movement
with the appropriate amount of effort. Once you
have found it, adjust the pace so that it feels soothing
to you. You are rocking your bones from the heels up
to the head. Let your whole body be floppy and let
the movement travel through you.

9 Let the movement stop. Rest.

10 Notice how your whole body rests on the floor, and
notice how your bones rest. Does it feel different
from when you started? The floor hasn't changed,
but your relationship to it has.

11 Start it again and let it go. Each time you do this
movement, let yourself tune into the sensation of
doing nothing, as a contrast to the jiggling. What do
you let go of? Do you notice that you feel that more
of you is on the floor?

12 Bring your awareness again to the back of the head,
the neck, upper and mid-back to your lower back
and pelvis: do they sit differently in their relationship
to the floor?

13 Notice how you breathe: what are you thinking of?
How are you feeling? Notice how you might feel a
sense of muscle contractions having dissolved. You
might also notice that your body feels awakened and
is perhaps even fizzing with a sensation that makes
you aware of your whole self, from your fingertips to
your toes.

Make this your daily practice—especially before you go to
bed—to reorganize your systems and release the tension in
your body.

What you have learned in this chapter

- Human beings are a complex interwoven network
  of systems. Whether you realize it or not, you are
  in a relationship with your whole self: you can
  decide to make that relationship either fractious or
  compassionate.
- Your nervous system is in a continuous iterative
  communication loop to and from the body. The
  experiences you feed it will determine how you

feel and how you interact with others and your
environment.

- Your nervous system has "go" and "no-go" functions.
  In our modern lives we tend to favor the "go" part,
  but we need to balance it with equal emphasis on the
  "no-go" function.
- Your brain is predictive rather than reactive. Its
  predictions are based on prior experience, which is
  confirmed or corrected by sensory input that forms
  maps in the brain of your body in its environment.
- If you want to make changes to your life, then you
  need to consider the master system—your nervous
  system—and feed it new experiences to draw from.

In the next chapter you will learn about the different senses
that influence your brain and the rest of your nervous system.

2

Body Sensing

In order to change, people need to become aware of
their sensations and the way that their bodies interact
with the world around them. Physical self-awareness
is the first step in releasing the tyranny of the past.

Bessel van der Kolk, *The Body Keeps the Score*

Have you ever been in conversation with someone and, without looking up, you sensed there was a stranger listening in
behind you? Perhaps you could feel their stillness and you
could picture one ear cocked toward you. Or you have had
the notion of someone you know being untruthful, because
their manner was a bit off? You sensed that they were being
inauthentic, but couldn't describe in words why you felt
that. You just had an innate knowledge somewhere in your
belly that they were being untrue.

It's these bodily sensations that we sometimes experience—
before we can describe the feeling—that we are going to
explore in this chapter; these senses that seem to sit underneath the layer of language. In the last chapter we looked
at how the senses are honed when you are in the womb,
learning about your environment and differentiating your
boundaries from those of your mother; feeling, sensing, and

being moved by your mother, which allows you to form in a relational way, to define yourself in relationship to your mother and as a separate entity from her.

When you are born, you are still a work in progress— your wiring instructions are gathered from the world around you through your body, and through your sense data. You learn how to read your mother's reactions and respond by mirroring them. Infants are sensitive to facial expression, tone of voice, posture, pace of movement, incipient action and physiological changes.[1] You form your experiences of the world pre-language, and in relationship with your caregiver. How they attune to you in your early years influences how you learn to self-regulate, along with your body temperature, levels of comfort and social interactions with others.

If your caregiver picked you up as soon as you cried, you probably felt safe. As you grow into an adult, you will be comfortable showing others that you are upset. You probably don't feel you must always put on a brave front and are able to display the full spectrum of what it means for you to be your whole self. However, if you got scolded every time you cried or were ignored, you may not want to show any feelings that are not positive, in case it means that you lose approval or, even worse, are ignored. If you experience adversity over a prolonged period, your brain will predict future periods of adversity based on your experience in the past.

You don't unlearn things, but you can learn new things. Exposure to those new things will reduce the influence of the old experiences. You can cultivate new experiences that feed your brain to predict differently in the future, to widen your library of predictions. Not being able to listen in to your bodily sensations leaves you in a state of cognitive dissonance where you *think* you have left past experiences behind and are living in the moment; however, you might *feel* something entirely different.

Being able to tune into your senses and respond accordingly enables you to fully inhabit your body and your mind.

Case study: Mary

One of my clients, Mary, came to me feeling broken and unsure of herself. She was in her late fifties and was living without a partner for the first time in her adult life. Her second husband, it transpired, had had numerous affairs throughout their fifteen-year marriage. The signs were there, but she always believed his protestations. He would shower her with presents and holidays, which Mary realized were an unspoken apology of sorts. The final straw came when she found out that her husband had fathered a child with another woman, with whom he had been in a relationship for six years. Mary was naturally devastated and, when she came to me, wanted to understand how she could get over his betrayal.

She wasn't sleeping, she found getting through the day hard going, she was often tearful or angry. She would often find herself gasping for breath and felt anxious about the future. Physically she held herself tightly, as if she wanted to curl in on herself. She had to keep it together for her job and for her teenage daughter, who was also dealing with feelings of abandonment by her father. Mary had to bear the brunt of her daughter's anguish, which was often directed against her, and felt she had no one she could turn to. She had a senior position in a precarious industry and it was important to her, and financially necessary, to keep everything going, even though she wanted to get into bed and, as she put it, never get up again.

We worked together to gently explore Mary's physical holding patterns and got her to be curious about her sensations, feelings, and thoughts. The beauty of this practice is that you don't have to talk about your problems and issues, or try to problem-solve using your mind. You simply allow your body to notice its holding patterns, and this awareness creates new choices—to hold these patterns or to let them go? How does it feel to let go of them? Once you consciously release them, you feel lighter and more open. You have now introduced this new possibility of how you could be if you were not holding on to this tension pattern. You cultivate an awareness of when you feel comfort and when you feel discomfort. This seems obvious, but often we don't feel anything at all until we feel pain or hit a wall with exhaustion. Over time and with practice, this new awareness restores balance to your nervous system because you are moving away from predictive reactions and instead learn to tune in to how you feel, not how you *tell* yourself you feel. You learn to be fully embodied with your whole self by listening; you are no longer in an ongoing conflict between your body and mind.

In our sessions, Mary learned to attend to her breathing to improve her brain function, so that she could make decisions from a calmer and more considered place. She slowly learned how to let go of the physical patterns she had knotted herself into, because her body knew that her partner had lied to her for most of their marriage, but her mind had hoped it wasn't so. When I guided her in our sessions, I observed that whenever she couldn't interpret my guidance into movement or she found something challenging, her fingers would curl into her palms, making fists. She had never noticed that.

If you think back to the tensegrity principle (see page 38), you might remember that tension in one place will influence the whole structure; in this case, Mary's external body-tensing had an effect on the quality of her breathing and her ability to release muscle tension. Learning something new is more difficult if you are in "doing" mode, as your brain can only process new movement and concepts if it isn't also having to deal with tension (and possibly danger), which uses up valuable resources.

With regular practice, Mary was able to bring awareness to the quality of her fingers. Over time, this new awareness helped her to shift her idea of herself as the weak, gullible, and heartbroken person who initially came to me, into someone who could survive this tumultuous event in her life. She reminded herself of all the other things she had endured and moved on from: getting a good degree, even though she had to pay her own way through college; the difficult birth of her daughter; a demanding job and her first divorce. She also shifted from feeling undeserving of her husband's love to righteous anger toward him. This gave her permission to genuinely feel her feelings, which stoked the fire to build a new and different life with her daughter.

All it took for Mary to change her self-image was cultivating awareness of her current situation, reorganizing, and then acting, based on this new information. Doesn't that make you feel hopeful? That changing your self-image is so much simpler than you thought.

Tuning in

Learning to soothe starts with learning to feel, which starts with sensing what is going on physically, in your body, and interpreting these sensations into emotions from a place of calm and safety. You begin to tune in to the signals that your body gives you: whether there is any tension in your neck, for example. You can also develop your attunement skills, which means that you become more aware of your own heartbeat, for instance, or sense how the breath travels into your body as you inhale. This deep connection to your feeling state enables you to begin to care more deeply for yourself.

Awareness is the first step in soothing your nervous system. How does your nervous system process these sensations or sense data? If your nervous system is soothed by tuning in to your senses, why doesn't it tune in to them automatically? It may seem like a good idea to be able to listen automatically to your internal body signals, but if you noticed all your sensations, there wouldn't be any headspace to do the things you actively want to do. There wouldn't be space to be creative, to understand complex concepts or even to go on wild adventures. Above all, tuning in to internal sensations could easily turn into self-denial and austerity, and where's the joy in that?

However, it is useful at times to be able to tune in to specific bodily sensations (your interoceptive sense), as this enables you to become more aware of your physical and emotional state. It can help you make better decisions about your health and well-being and cope with stress more effectively. You will be able to regulate your emotions better and avoid feeling overwhelmed by them, and make better choices when you are feeling stressed or upset. You will be able to avoid or prevent injury, as you will know when to take a rest or realize that an activity is dangerous and stop doing it. If your tendency is to work all hours and you don't know how to break the cycle of filling your time with more work, you will come to a realization of this.

With awareness of your body's signals, you can make adjustments to your behavior to improve the quality of your life. For example, if you are feeling tired, you can take a break in order to rest. Or if you are feeling stressed, you can take some deep breaths to calm down. If your neck is sore from being hunched over your laptop, it is time to move out of that position. If you feel short-tempered because you are tired, you can plan a better sleep routine. If you stare at the screen uninterrupted for hours on end and your eyes are dry and tired, you can introduce regular eye movements. The signs are always there, so why do we not listen in and take appropriate action when we feel out of sorts? What drives us to work all hours? To stay up late watching Netflix, when we are tired? Why do we not look after ourselves?

My clients give many reasons as to why they do not commit to caring for themselves. Often they place themselves at the bottom of their list of priorities, because there are other people to tend to. They find ways to distract themselves from their problems as a means of coping with stress. They are bored or restless, or they procrastinate from getting on with a job that feels daunting. You also have to keep in mind that streaming series and social media are designed to tantalize you and keep you hooked and, before you know it, it's the early hours of the morning. Initially it takes an enormous amount of willpower to commit to noticing your habits and forming new ones.

It is important to remember that chronic conditions start from small, unattended niggles and tension. To prevent this happening, it is vital to pause and notice where you are; to consider how you feel and, if you are in discomfort, tend to yourself with appropriate action. While working long hours is sometimes necessary, doing this all the time isn't sustainable and will have an impact on your long-term health and enjoyment of life. You are not a machine that can keep going for hours, day in and day out, without consequences for your health. Listening to your bodily signals will help you manage your energy and your well-being.

Case study: Layla

Layla was referred to me by her psychotherapist, who didn't know how to continue to support her client. Layla experienced somatic system disorder (SSD), a mental-health condition in which someone experiences physical symptoms that cannot be explained by a medical condition. The symptoms can be severe and disabling, often leading to significant distress and anxiety. SSD is thought to be caused by a combination of factors, including trauma (such as physical or sexual abuse), neglect, or war. Dissociation is also a mental process that allows someone to detach from their thoughts, feelings, or memories. It is a common coping mechanism for people who have experienced trauma.

The symptoms of SSD can vary from person to person, but they may include pain that isn't caused by an injury or medical condition; numbness or tingling in the hands, feet, or other parts of the body; blurred or double vision; changes in sleep patterns, such as difficulty in sleeping or sleeping too much; and, as in Layla's case, seizures that would leave her feeling upset, anxious, and depleted for the rest of the day. We didn't talk about what had happened to her—I don't need to know anything the client doesn't want to share. But I can observe where someone is holding their body in a protective pattern that inhibits their breathing or movement. If Layla was surprised by something, it had the potential to trigger a seizure, so she often felt hyper-alert to everything that was happening in her environment.

Bessel van der Kolk,[2] a psychiatrist and trauma expert, says that traumatized people who cannot feel subtle sensations often become drawn to dangerous situations and pursuits because they seek stimulation. They have lost the ability to feel safe and comfortable in their bodies. He explains that when we experience trauma, our brains go into a state of hyper-arousal. This means that we are constantly alert for danger and our bodies are flooded with stress hormones. As a result, we may become hypersensitive to stimuli, even to things that do not usually bother us. Over time, this hyper-arousal can lead to a desensitization of our bodies. We may become numb to physical sensations, including pain, pleasure, and hunger. To feel something, traumatized people may seek out dangerous situations and pursuits. These activities can provide a temporary sense of excitement and aliveness, but can also be harmful. For example, someone who is numb to pain may engage in self-harm, while someone who is numb to pleasure may become addicted to drugs or alcohol.

Layla was drawn to fast sports and she watched thrillers as entertainment, even though both of these had the potential to trigger a seizure. When we started to work together, we looked at simple movements to make her feel safe and comfortable in her body. We also explored the sensations that told her she was about to go into a seizure. We explored where she felt her breathing in her body, and the difference between contracted and released muscle tension. This helped Layla to expand her "window of tolerance"—the range of emotional arousal that someone can comfortably manage. When we are within our window of toler-ance we are able to feel our emotions without becoming over-whelmed or dysregulated; when we are outside our window of tolerance, we may experience difficulty regulating our emotions, which can lead to anxiety, depression, or anger. People with a history of trauma or neglect may have a narrower window of toler-ance than those who have not experienced these things.

After our sixth session Layla could stop a seizure from taking hold, because she could sense the feelings that lead to a seizure, her chest tightening and her breath getting faster. By the last session Layla felt calmer at rest, and she was confident that she could "read" her body to ensure that a seizure would not take hold. She removed stressors from her life, because she now had a felt sense of calmness. Instead of spinning classes and mountain biking she added yoga and tai chi to her repertoire of practices to calm her system. She left with simple, soothing movements to practice when she felt the alarm sensations that typically led to a seizure, plus a library of all our sessions, ready to practice whenever she needed to reset her system.

The question is: *when* is it useful to listen in to your bodily signals? To answer that, it is helpful to understand the main task of your brain, which is a part of your nervous system. As you know, it is the job of your brain to budget the resources for your body.[3] Your brain needs to predict how much of those resources you need for your actions *before* you need it. If your body doesn't get the resources in good time, there will be a price to pay.

The most resource-heavy activities that you can engage in

are movement and learning new things. When you don't get enough resources to do these things, then your metabolism—the process of converting food to energy—isn't as efficient as it should be. This results in feeling fatigued and you might have to stop moving so much to conserve your energy. You then experience uncomfortable feelings that come up when you are not moving very much, such as tightness or soreness of your muscles.

Because your muscles are tense from lack of movement, your sleep will be affected and this in turn may lead to you feeling that your problems are insurmountable, because you are so tired. Your physical and mental tension will influence your day: a tired brain remembers negative experiences, but forgets positive ones.[4] Your brain uses about 20 percent of your resources.[5] An energy-efficient strategy for your brain, when faced with any situation, is to reassemble your past experiences to figure out quickly how much energy to use for this experience. If it tries to learn about every experience that you encounter, it can cost you time—time that you might need to get away from a threat. Your brain tries to learn from your experiences to reduce uncertainty; it predicts what is going to happen next and allocates the right resources for this event, because if it didn't, there might be dire consequences, and even death. Thinking, seeing, and feeling are all in service to keeping you alive and well.

Let's pause here to take in this information, because to me it is mind-blowing. Your brain is making continuous calculations based on your experiences, and is confirming or refining its experience with the sense data coming from your body. You are not meeting events in the moment they are happening; you are assembling your previously learned responses, asking yourself, "What is this most like?" and then throwing out your response to meet the moment. This is necessary for your survival. However, if you want to change how you respond, or alter your behavior, then listening in to the signals from your body will help you disrupt your automatic responses.

Let's explore this concept with an example. Perhaps when you were young you were repeatedly told that you were stupid—maybe your teacher told you this, or perhaps it was a parent. You heard it so often that it became your belief, and you even say it to yourself whenever you get things wrong. Now, in your adult life, this idea about yourself makes you reticent to put up your hand to answer questions or to speak in public, even though you are no longer a child. In work meetings, your face burns with shame at the thought of not having the right answer to a problem, and you dread anyone looking at you. Your hands feel sweaty at the thought of being put on the spot. Even though conceptually you know that you can do challenging things, inwardly you still feel like a child who is hardwired to get things wrong. Your racing mind is your brain trying to make sense of the sensations in your body. You know that you are no longer a child, but your nervous system is experiencing the same sensations that you once felt and it feels confusing to you.

How should you address this? If you pause, breathe, and reassess the situation, you can tune in to your current sensory information. And you can cultivate more curiosity about your sensations: could they be more about your *physical* discomfort? Perhaps the office heating is too high; perhaps you didn't sleep and are tired, and this lies behind your physical sensation. Being curious about this saves you from the relentless emotional suffering that is brought about by thinking that you are not good enough and cannot cope. Now that you have minimized the feeling of unworthiness to a bodily sensation, you can tend to the physical discomfort. Once you do that, you learn to calm your nervous system so that you don't feel alarmed every time someone asks you a question. You learn to override the impulse from your past, by feeding new experiences to your nervous system. This gives it a wider choice of predictions. You now have more options about what assumptions your brain makes.

What happens if you don't listen in? You stay in this disconnected place where you are in a constant battle with an overthinking mind and a body that is exhausted with ongoing tension. There is a different way to live, and it starts by cultivating a more compassionate relationship with yourself.

Your body sends sense data-streams to your nervous system—you can also call these sensations "feelings"—and these are interpreted into your emotions. Your emotions influence your thoughts, and your thoughts will influence your actions, and over time your actions become your behaviors. From this, you can see why it is important to disrupt the predictions that your brain makes, and you can do this using "embodiment" or "somatic awareness."[6]

How does this play out in a live situation? I used to hate speaking to camera, as I only ever saw the things that looked wrong. I pull funny faces, I start my sentences with "So . . . ," I look tired, and I don't want to be judged and criticized. It's interesting to me that I can easily get up and teach a crowd of hundreds, but talking about *what* I do, rather than just doing it, used to bring about an existential crisis for me every time.

Behavior

↑

Actions

↑

Thoughts

↑

Emotions

↑

Sensations

Sense data-streams

Video content is an important part of marketing my
work, so I decided to take the emotion out of it. I breathed
and soothed my physical body, and made a conscious decision to put aside comparisons with what everyone else was
doing and just get on with it. I ensured that my setup made
me feel physically comfortable. The camera had to be at the
right distance and not too close to my face. I prefer to stand
when I am talking, so that I allow the natural movement
in my body to flow. I filmed myself again and again and
watched the videos back, to see what worked and what didn't
work in terms of angles, what I was wearing, where I placed
the camera, and so on. I also made the decision that it was
important that I show myself as a human being, rather than
as a perfect, idealized version of myself, as that wouldn't
chime with what I teach. Once I realized that I needed to feel

physically comfortable and made this my priority, speaking to camera didn't cause me such anxiety anymore.

Let's now look at the senses, to understand the sources of information from the body to the brain and how you can interpret them. Some of the senses will be familiar to you, but there may be a couple that you are less aware of.

Vision

When you consider your visual system you probably think about viewing the world through your eyes. Your visual system, however, is more than simply seeing. This system signals whether it is day or night and is critical to the brain and the rest of your bodily systems. The visual system also governs your mood, level of alertness, sleep, and appetite.[7] It takes up almost half of the space in your brain, which implies that it has a far-reaching influence on the rest of your body.

Our eyes are part of our central nervous system. When we develop in the womb, two pieces of our brain are pushed out of our skull and form our eyes, which are in effect part of our brain, but sit outside the skull.

The job of the eyes is to collect light information and send it to the rest of the brain through the retinas. These are the parts of the eyes that convert light into neural signals. You might remember, from school biology, that you have photoreceptors that help you to see at dusk and in mono-chrome, and ones that allow you to see in daylight and in color permutations of red, blue, and green. The light is converted into electrical information that is sent off to the rest of the brain via other specialized cells.

Through lightning-speed calculations, everything that you see is not what you see directly, but is a best guess based on the pattern of electricity received by your brain. Imagine that you are looking at a red flower: the photoreceptors that respond best to the light bouncing off the red flower enable you to perceive it as red. It does this by comparing the amount of red that comes off the flower with the green and blue around it. The light information is transformed into electrical signals that your visual system understands. It is the comparison of these signals that allows you to understand what color the flower is.

But it isn't only with colors that your brain does quick-fire calculations to make sense of the world. The brain makes guesses based on your visual impression of what you see in your environment. For instance, information coming into the eye is in two dimensions, so the brain must work out the world in terms of depth, and it does this with the knowledge that has been gained by your life experience of learning. When you look at a building in the distance, it appears smaller in contrast to the buildings closer to you—your brain does the calculation for you based on your experience to allow you to understand that you are looking at a building in the distance and not at a tiny house.

Aside from sight, the visual system's primary purpose is to inform your brain and body of where you are in terms of day or night. Whether you feel sleepy or awake, your pain threshold, how fast your metabolism is—all this is rooted in time, based on where the earth is in relation to the sun.

However, we are spending more and more of our time looking at our screens, rather than outside or looking into the distance. The average US adult spends 6,259 hours a year staring at screens—be that a phone, a laptop, a gaming device, or a television—and this equates to forty-four years over a lifetime.[8] The ability to carry your screen around with you wherever you go is a recent phenomenon, and you can now shop for groceries in the post-office line and read about civil unrest somewhere across the world while lying in your bed. There seems to be no respite for your eyes or, indeed, for your brain.

How does fixing your eyes on something close to you, like a phone, affect your eyes, and how does it influence your bodily systems? In quite surprising ways, it turns out.

The lens of your eye enables you to focus on objects at varying distances. In a process called accommodation, your lens moves dynamically to make it thicker and thinner according to what you are looking at and whether it is close to you or farther away. This movement also influences the tiny muscles in the eye that move the lens, by bringing a blood supply to the muscles and to the neurons (nerve cells) that are responsible for focusing the lens. When the lens loses this elasticity, your close-up vision is impaired. But that is not all. Where your eyes focus is also where your attention goes, which will have an influence on your mental alertness. Inhibiting the movement of the eyes—keeping the lens fixed—uses energy, which is one of the reasons that sitting looking at a screen all day can make you feel fatigued. Healthy pupils dilate when you look at something far away and contract when you look at something nearby.

Spending most of your time indoors and focusing on objects close to you is unhealthy for your eyes; it shapes the neural circuitry of the eyes to stay fixed. Not getting sunlight early in the day, to activate the wakefulness processes of the bodily systems, and having your eyes fixed close will affect your well-being. When you look far away at the horizon, this is one of the best ways to relax your visual system and is something that I frequently practice and recommend to my clients.

As human beings, we evolved outdoors, yet our modern lifestyles necessitate us being indoors during the day, generally in lower levels of light. We then extend the day beyond dusk with artificial light and devices. This shift in lifestyle lies behind the increasing rate of myopia, or shortsightedness, in children, causing blurred distance vision. Our lifestyles, it would seem, are not conducive to living optimally. However, recent trials show that getting at least two hours of daylight every day reduces the chances of myopia, so all is not lost.[9] Understanding what your system needs to function well will enable you to create routines in your day that will help you to thrive.

Vision lesson

Try these simple techniques:

1   Take a break from your computer every thirty minutes either by going outside or by throwing open a window and looking at the horizon. Panoramic viewing allows the eyes to relax.

2   It is also important to retrain your eye to look at different depths of vision. Try this near–far viewing outside: hold a finger up at arm's length and focus your eyes on it. Slowly move your finger toward you and allow your eyes to refocus on it, so that your

eyes are about to cross but don't go there; then move your finger away and keep focusing on it as it moves away from you. Repeat this a few times. This will help to offset nearsightedness.

Smell

Your olfactory sense is one of the first to develop, before vision and hearing. Your nose is part of your respiratory system and is responsible for smell. When you smell something by sniffing, the smell enters your nose as a chemical and gets captured by the specific receptor-type in your brain. Your brain has forty million different olfactory receptor neurons.[10] Your olfactory bulb is a collection of neurons right above the roof of your mouth, and these neurons extend out of the skull into the nostrils and respond to different odors. Smell goes straight to your brain.

Scent and your survival are inextricably linked to each other. When you smell a fire, you need to either get away or put it out; either way, this type of smell requires your immediate action. If you detect the smell of rotten food, you know not to eat it because it will make you ill. These smells go straight to the fear- and threat-detection part of your brain, the amygdala.

There are also odors that make you want to move toward them: think about how you feel when you smell chocolate or freshly baked bread. Some pathways are linked with an association that you have learned; it could be that the jasmine perfume your grandmother wore means that every time you smell jasmine, it will always be intertwined with your memories of her. We also sense ourselves and our boundaries—such as the smells in our home, the familiar scents of our partner, our family and the food we eat. We can also detect strange smells in our surroundings: if a stranger has been in the house, or if something unfamiliar has been delivered at the front door. My husband wears an aftershave oil that he puts on when we are going out, and it has the fragrance oud as an ingredient. Whenever I smell it, an involuntary smile forms on my face, as it means we are going out to have a good time.

Sniffing and inhalation have positive effects on the way you acquire and retain information. When you inhale, you increase your brain's alertness and attention. Inhaling is a cue for the brain to pay attention and wakes it up. Sniffing as an action has a powerful effect on focus and information retention. Interestingly, nasal-breathers learn better than mouth-breathers, or those with a combination of nasal and mouth breathing.[11] If you have no issues with breathing through your nose, then training yourself to do so will have a positive and immediate effect on your health.

Smell lesson

1   Gather something that you like the smell of. It could be your favorite perfume, an essential oil, a warming spice or a fruit.
2   Find a quiet place where you will not be disturbed.
3   Sit comfortably and close your eyes. Take a deep breath out and, as you gently breathe in, waft the item underneath your nose. Notice what you feel in your nose and throat. Notice the skin on your face and the hairs on the back of your neck.

4 Where else can you "feel" the smell? What emotions
   or memories come up for you?

5 Take the item away from your nose and sit with that
   feeling for a few breaths. When you are done, slowly
   open your eyes.

Taste

Taste is so much more than a product of your taste buds
on your tongue. Taste is a combination of how food looks,
smells, tastes, and feels in the mouth. You would expect a
raw carrot to have a crunch and a sweetness to it and, if it
didn't, you might think it had gone off. Your tongue can
taste sweet, sour, salty, bitter, and umami, which has a meaty,
brothy taste and fat content. Your taste receptors are organized along your tongue. Your sweet receptors respond to
sugars, and your salty receptors respond to salt. The gus-
tatory nerve travels from the tongue to the region of your
brain called the insular cortex, which serves as a hub for
sensory, emotional, motivational, socialization, and cognitive
systems, where the tastes are organized.[12] You can recognize
taste in a rapid 100 milliseconds. Sweet tastes signal a rapid
energy source, salty tastes signal sodium and bitter receptors
signal spoiled food.

Your taste neurons sit under the tongue's surface and
regenerate within a week. Taste is broken down and chemical signals are interpreted from the food that you eat. Taste
receptors are not only found on your tongue; you also have
taste receptors in your gut, your digestive system and your
reproductive organs. If you remember from the last chapter,
we saw that the three layers formed in the early embryo give

rise to your cells and tissues. The innermost layer gives rise to the digestive tract, respiratory tract, and urinary tract, and the middle layer gives rise to muscles, bones, blood, the circulatory system, and your reproductive organs. There is often a sensual element to eating and tasting delicious tastes, so could there be a remembered relationship in the tissues themselves? Those who work with the mind and body as an integrated system would argue that there might be something in this.

Genetics play a part in your sense of taste, as does your environment. How you perceive taste will be different from how I perceive taste. How well you can smell, or taste things, is often a good indication of your brain health. Taste buds have a short life and turn over within a matter of days, and this slows down as you get older, so you might find that you need to add more sugar or salt to get the same taste.

Taste lesson

1   Gather a few pieces of food that you like to eat, choosing a few different tastes.
2   Close your eyes and take a few deep breaths.
3   Take the first piece of food to your nose and give it a gentle sniff. What happens in your mouth? Place a small piece of this food on your tongue. Focus on the sensations in your mouth as you let it sit on your tongue.
4   Notice the texture of the food: is it smooth, rough, spiky, sticky, or does it melt? What is the texture as you bite into it?
5   Once you have swallowed it, pay attention to the aftereffects of the food: how does it make you feel?

6 Drink some water to cleanse your palate before your move on to the next taste. Pay attention to the different flavors of the food, such as its sweetness, sourness, saltiness, bitterness, or umami flavor. And notice the different smells of the food, as they can also affect your sense of taste.

7 Once you have finished tasting the food, open your eyes and think about how the different sensations and flavors made you feel.

Hearing

Your ability to hear sounds requires both your ear and your brain. Your ear receives the sound, and your brain makes sense of it. The ear is a complex organ that is responsible for hearing and balance. It is divided into three parts: the outer ear, the middle ear and the inner ear.

The outer ear is responsible for collecting sound waves and funneling them into the ear canal, which is a narrow tube that leads to the eardrum. The eardrum is a thin membrane that vibrates when sound waves hit it.

The middle ear is responsible for amplifying sound waves and sending them to the inner ear. The middle ear contains three tiny bones called the malleus, incus, and stapes. These bones are connected to each other and to the eardrum. When the eardrum vibrates, it causes the bones to vibrate as well. This amplification helps to make sounds louder. You will also find the facial nerve here, which moves the muscle in your face, and a nerve responsible for taste.

The inner ear is responsible for converting sound waves into nerve signals that are sent to the brain. It contains a spiral-shaped organ called the cochlea, which is filled with fluid and contains tiny hair cells. When sound waves hit the cochlea, they cause the fluid to move. This movement bends the hair cells, which sends nerve signals to the brain, which then interprets these signals as sound.

The ear also plays a role in balance. The inner ear contains a structure called the vestibular system, which is responsible for detecting movement and orientation. It helps us to keep our balance and to know where we are in space, and when we are moving through space.

There are many stop-off points from the ear to the brain, because it is crucial to our survival to know which direction a sound is coming from—whether near or far. You have neurons in your brain that calculate whether the sound is coming from the right or the left ear. The outer structure of your ears also gives you information about whether the sound is coming from above. A small muscle in your inner ear contracts when there is an ongoing loud noise, to protect your inner ear from damage.

Patterns of what the sound is, and where it is in space, are worked out according to which ear the sound is perceived by. Auditory information goes into your cortex, which is responsible for higher-level planning. Your visual system is mapped to areas in your brain, as is your auditory system. The auditory cortex is located in the temporal lobe at the sides of the brain. It is responsible for processing auditory information and making sense of it. The auditory cortex is organized in a way that reflects the manner in which sounds are organized in the real world. For example, high-frequency sounds are processed in the front of the auditory cortex, while low-frequency sounds are processed in the back.

You can expand or contract your auditory awareness; you can tune out all the noise in background chatter and focus on the person near you. Similar to panoramic vision, you can expand or limit the sounds around you. Using this attentional system, you can access neuroplasticity, the adult brain's ability to change, reorganize, or grow neural networks.

Your balance and spatial awareness are influenced and regulated by your vestibular system. This is made up of three semicircular canals, which are arranged at ninety-degree angles to each other, and of the two otolith organs, which detect linear acceleration, gravitational force and tilting movements.

Your vestibular system works closely with your visual system to inform you about your space and position. The mechanisms in your inner ear inform your eyes where to travel, and at the same time your visual system informs your vestibular system which way up you are, and which way you are turned relative to your environment.

Because we spend so much time sitting down or staying in one position, our ability to balance has been hugely impacted. You have probably heard that standing on one leg can improve your body and brain communication and is a marker of longevity. When you stand on one leg you are taking in signals from your visual system, your vestibular system and your proprioceptive system in the muscles, joints, and tendons. Wobbling and recalibrating these systems is a good way to connect your bones, joints, muscles, skin, eyes, and ears to work together. Your proprioceptive sensors are in a feedback loop with your brain and your motor nerves, to negotiate your balance in gravity.

Moving slowly is challenging for both your vestibular

system and your visual system. Tilting, leaning in, and unstable surfaces are all great challenges for your balance.

Hearing lesson

1 Sit down with your feet on the floor.
2 Let your eyes close. Breathe in and out of your nose.
3 Open up your ears as if they are microphones and let all the noises float in.
4 Start to tune in to the noises in your environment: the clicking of your radiators, the running of water, the noises of people in your building, birds singing outside, the sound of the rain on your window, and so on.
5 Begin to turn your ears to the sound that is farthest away. Take your time to do this, then attune your ears to the sound that is second-farthest away, and keep going until you arrive at the sound that is closest to you. Pause on each sound for a few breaths before you move on.
6 Let it all go.
7 Now attune to the sound that is closest to you and travel your awareness out to the sound that is farthest away from you. Pause on each sound before you move on to the next one.
8 Bring your attention from outward to inward sounds one more time. Let it go.
9 Breathe in and out a few times with your eyes closed. When you are done, slowly open your eyes and notice how you feel.

Touch

There is a deep biological connection between your sense of touch and your emotional state. Tactile communication involves a complex system processed by the skin, which is made up of billions of nerve cells. These send signals to the region of your brain called the somatosensory cortex, which makes sense of the touch data: is it a friendly touch? Is it slow or fast? What are the temperature and pressure? Do you move toward it or away from it?

The neurons on the skin respond to specific stimuli, such as pressure, and send these as an electrical signal to the somatosensory cortex via the spinal cord. The somatosensory cortex is responsible for processing information about touch, pressure, temperature, and pain. It is organized in a way that reflects the relative sensitivity of different parts of the body. The areas of the body that are most sensitive—such as the hands, fingertips, lips, tongue, nose, eyes, genitals, and feet—have a much larger representation in the somatosensory cortex than the parts of the body that are less sensitive, such as the back and the arms. This is because the brain has more neurons dedicated to processing signals from the more sensitive parts of the body, which enables us to get a more detailed and accurate perception of these areas.

Your brain interprets the information coming from your sensory nerves and sends out impulses through your motor nerves to allow you to take the appropriate action. As a reminder, your brain contextualizes the sense data by anticipation, anxiety, and interpretation of what is happening, which drives your perception of what is occurring.[13]

Friendly touch has been shown to calm the effects of stress—holding the hand of a loved one dials down the stress response when they are going through a demanding experience.[14] In another study, premature newborns who received three sessions daily of fifteen-minute touch therapy for five to ten days gained 47 percent more weight than preterm babies who followed standard treatment.[15]

You may remember soothing yourself when you were a child. Perhaps you had a tantrum and, because you were once rocked by your mother, you learned to rock yourself to a calmer state. The way we soothed ourselves when we were younger will still work to soothe us as adults, because our nervous system has the same structure. The difference is that, in the process of living, we've added layers of life experience to our nervous system that keep us in a more hypervigilant state than when our caregivers looked after everything.

Touch lesson

1   Warm up your hands by rubbing them together. Let your eyes close.

2   Place one hand at the top of your breastbone and stroke it down to the bottom of your breastbone, and let the other hand stroke from the top of your breastbone to the bottom, so that you always have one hand on your breastbone: one strokes downward, followed by the other, as if you were stroking a cat with both hands.

3   Tune into the sensations on your hands and your breastbone. Let your breathing be even.

4   Do this a few times and, once you stop, keep your eyes closed and notice how you feel.

Proprioception

Have you ever wondered how you know where your arm is, without looking at it? Or how you know where you are in space, without having to look around? This is all down to *proprioception*, the ability to sense where your body is in space using tiny sensors in your muscles, skin, and joints.

Proprioceptors are specialized sensory receptors that send signals to the brain about the position, movement, and tension of your body parts. These signals help you to maintain balance, coordinate movement, and perceive your body's position in space.

Proprioception is a complex process that involves the integration of information from multiple sources, including proprioceptors, vision, and vestibular input (from the inner ear). It is essential for many activities, including walking, running, dancing, and playing sports. It is also important for activities of daily living, such as dressing and eating. Proprioception can be affected by a number of factors, including injury and disease, and when you stop including balance, coordination and non-habitual movement as part of your daily routine, as you get older. When proprioception is impaired, it can lead to problems with balance, coordination, and movement. Proprioception is an important part of our overall sense of self, enabling us to move through the world safely and confidently.

Proprioception lesson

1   To feel your proprioceptive sense in action, come to a standing position. Pick up one leg to balance on your supporting leg, allowing this knee to bend slightly.

2 Let the toes of the standing leg be long—don't
   scrunch them up—and gently press your big toe,
   little toe and the center of your heel into the floor.
   Most people should be able to do this.
3 Tune in to the sensations that you feel in your hip,
   knee, ankle, and across the bones of your feet. Can
   you feel the work going on to keep you balanced on
   one leg?
4 Now close your eyes. Most people will wobble
   and fall off-balance at this point. If you can stay
   balanced for ten seconds, you are doing well. If you
   are able to stay balanced with your eyes closed, did
   you notice how much more your whole body had to
   work to try to find your balance?

Achieving balance doesn't mean being rigid. Finding balance
requires the brain to create new neural connections. This is
because balance is a complex skill that integrates information from various sensory systems, such as your vestibular
system, visual system, and proprioceptive system. When you
take away one of those systems—your visual sense—then
your other systems have to work harder.

As you learn to balance, your brain constantly adjusts
how you move and shifts your body to keep you upright. This
process entails creating new neural connections between
different parts of the brain. With time, these connections
become more robust and more efficient, making it easier for
you to balance. Moreover, balance training can also enhance
your cognitive function. Focusing your attention and making
quick decisions can improve your memory, processing speed,
and problem-solving abilities.

So if you feel unsteady, don't worry. Remember that finding balance trains your brain to make new neural connections.

Interoception

This sense informs my work and it is attracting a lot of interest because cultivating it allows us to regulate our emotions and it is influenced by all the other senses.

To remind you, interoception is your brain's representation of the sensations from your body. Your brain's task is to regulate the internal systems by anticipating the needs of your body and delivering resources before you need them. Interoception is central to everything, from emotions and thought to your self-image.[16]

I have more than touched (sorry!) upon this sense in this chapter and will continue to do so elsewhere, so I won't say more here. Every lesson and practice in this book is an interoceptive exploration, and I'll let you take your pick of them from the many you'll find within it.

What you have learned in this chapter

- The eyes signal day or night, and influence all the other systems to wake up or to rest.
- The eyes also influence your mental focus, and the eye lens dynamically adjusts to what you are looking at.
- Your taste and smell are intertwined.
- Proprioception is an integration of many of your senses.
- Interoception—your ability to sense the signals from

your internal body—self-regulates your emotions and reduces levels of anxiety and stress.

- Living fully open to your senses will cultivate a more meaningful relationship with yourself.

In the next chapter we will explore the breath. This acts as a direct switch to your brain, so if you want to change your thoughts, change your breath first. We will look at how you can unlock your patterns of breathing to feel calm and organized.

3

The Breath

Breath is the bridge between your body and the universe.
Thich Nhat Hanh, Buddhist monk and peace activist,
Peace Is Every Step

Do you ever stop to think about your breathing? It's a strangely confrontational question, isn't it? Breathing is the very first thing you do when you enter existence as you are born, defining your life as a separate entity from your mother. It is the very last thing you do before you leave this earth. Yet we rarely stop to consider *how* we breathe.

How are you breathing right now? Did you hold your breath as your eyes traced the letters along the page? Are you inadvertently holding your stomach in and breathing into your chest? Do you know why you breathe? Or how many breaths you take in a lifetime?

The average person in the US takes between twelve and twenty breaths per minute.[1] Breathing in and out counts as one breath, and typically you breathe 23,000 times throughout the day. In some traditions it is thought that you only have so many breaths in your lifetime, which makes me want to make every single breath count.

I thought I knew all about the breath, because I had been

taught the importance of breathing in my various trainings over the years. I had learned and taught pranayama—a yogic term that describes shifting energy, or prana, around the body with breathwork. I had completed many yoga courses, plus advanced anatomy in movement, Pilates, and personal trainer courses. I had studied meditation and been on many mind-and-body intensive trainings.

And yet . . . until I formulated The Human Method—which The Soothe Program is a part of—my breathing was still a separate action from my movement, and I tended to use my breath to push down the whirring of my mind in a reactive response. I paid attention to my breath only when I felt stressed or couldn't sleep. I was in a push-pull relationship with meditation and breathwork, as if I were pretending to do something outwardly, but inwardly my mind was chaotic and unbelieving. I had a long-standing meditation practice, but the end results were hard fought and not always guaranteed. The peace of breathing at an even pace is what I had hoped the practice of meditation would give me.

In classes, yogic breathing was often noisy and didn't seem integrated with the breath and body. In Pilates you are encouraged to inhale through the nose and exhale through the mouth and to pull your belly inward from the external body. In fitness you are taught to exhale through the mouth on the effort, and it all seems mechanistic, like a separate practice that is disconnected from the action. The quality of your breath is a window into your mental state. Yet I often saw this same mind-body battle in practices that claimed to promote mind-body integration. Despite intellectually understanding the anatomy and benefits of breathing,

I didn't understand it in a *somatic* sense—from my lived experience in my body.

Meditation is portrayed as the ultimate mind-calming balm, but if you aren't aware of how your breath changes throughout your day, in response to what is happening to you—and, more importantly, how you *perceive* what is happening to you—then a meditation practice will be hard to sustain. How you breathe is a gauge of your mental turmoil, and you need to pay attention to it. In my years of teaching and from my own personal practice, I have found that breathwork is the most powerful and accessible place from which to start a contemplative practice. How you breathe will immediately influence how you feel and think.

My meditation practice went out the window when the Covid-19 pandemic hit. I was naturally in a heightened state of anxiety because of all the uncertainty. This was a new disease and the levels of contagion were unknown; it was like living in a disaster movie. All the things that help us regulate our nervous system were instantly taken away. Going outside for more than one hour was banned; gathering with friends and family, hugging one another, and even traveling into work and having casual conversations with colleagues or interactions with strangers. It was such an overwhelming experience of many emotions all at once, coupled with an underlying unease that our leaders would not be able to make the best decisions for us.

It was frightening to face possible death from something that no one had any prior knowledge of, and demoralizing to live with the possibility that the world we came back to afterward had learned zero lessons from the experience: that there seems to be limited will from above to reorganize to become a better, fairer, and more compassionate society.

There were hopeful signs that we could do things differently because we had the chance to pause and notice the world around us, and the outcome of people being forced to stay in one place and live much smaller lives allowed the natural world to flourish. There was less disruption to marine life; goats overran villages; roadkill rates went down and sea turtles got a boost in population, to cite just a few examples.[2] The reduction in pollution levels seemed to have a positive outcome for the health of the planet, if only temporarily.

Instead of doing a meditation practice to soothe my jangly brain, I spent a lot of time on the floor, rocking and breathing. Despite my best efforts, I would find myself glued to my phone, checking social media and searching for reliable news updates. Every time I heard something that sent me into anxiety and fear, I would rock them out of my system, which allowed me to release the muscles that held tension on hearing the unfolding news reports. The release of muscles enabled my body to accommodate my breath. Sitting still and trying to quiet my mind, however, didn't feel like a useful option for me in a time of such crisis.

Once you start to cultivate a conscious and slower breathing practice, the change will be immediate, which makes it compelling. Breathing consciously in and out is an easy practice to fit into your day. When you have a better understanding of your breath and how you can slow down your pace of breathing, a meditation practice becomes much easier to cultivate because you have already soothed your nervous system.

My clients range from athletes and time-pressed CEOs,

right through to those managing degenerative conditions such as Parkinson's disease. And regardless of their physical abilities, conscious breathing is the very first practice that I teach them. Conscious breathing comes first. How you breathe affects how you feel.

Case study: Phillip

I have a long-standing client named Phillip who has developed Parkinson's over the past few years. Parkinson's is a progressive nervous-system disorder that impacts on coordination and movement. Phillip is a highly successful businessman but, by his own admission, is one of the most un-self-aware people I have ever met. He has no language for his range of feelings and no understanding of the nuance of his feelings. I often ask him if he feels different from the state that he was in before he started his sessions with me. He generally has four responses: *yes, not sure, relaxed,* and *stretched*. But what is so refreshing about him is that he often questions why I ask him to do certain things. There is nothing better to sharpen one's teaching than a client who asks you "Why?" when you give them guidance. One of Phillip's questions to me was, "I am alive, which means that I am breathing, so why do I need to focus on my breathing?"

That's a great question.

Why do you breathe?

Breathing is instinctive—without it you would not be alive. You can live without food for about three weeks, without water for three days, but only for three minutes without oxygen. Every part of your body needs oxygen to survive.

Every function of your body, from thinking to digesting to moving, requires oxygen. When these metabolic processes take place, carbon dioxide is the waste product. You inhale to take in oxygen, which is delivered to the red blood cells and carried around the body, and you breathe out to get rid of carbon dioxide. Your blood has an optimal pH level—this defines whether the blood is more acidic or alkaline—and to maintain the pH level you need to get rid of the waste products.

Your nervous system, via the nerve cells in your body, sends electrical impulses to the brain stem to signal the amount of oxygen versus carbon dioxide in your blood. Your brain stem is the part of the brain connected to your spinal cord, and it deals with autonomic functions so that you don't have to think about them.

From these signals your brain stem sends a message to the muscles involved in breathing, your diaphragm—a dome-shaped muscle that sits underneath the lungs—as well as to the intercostals, the muscles in between your ribs. Your diaphragm contracts downward, enabling the lungs to increase in size, causing the internal air pressure to lower, which allows air from the outside to rush in. This is your inhale.

As you exhale, the diaphragm, ribs, and lungs recoil to their original position and air is expelled from the lungs. Oxygen being pulled in gets transferred to your bloodstream, while carbon dioxide is transferred into the air in your lungs, ready to be expelled. This signaling adjusts your breathing rate, dependent on how active you are and in order to restore the balance of blood pH.

So yes, breathing should be—and is—an instinctive

action. Your nervous system is designed simply for "go" or "no-go" (see page 34) to manage your energy. Yet our modern environment is highly stimulating and quite different from the one our ancestors lived in. We now have more potential stressors in our lives, because our nervous system cannot distinguish between a loud bang that we need to run away from and the relentless stream of information that we have to contend with. Added to that, we are likely to be more sedentary, passively receiving the potential stressors rather than acting to dissipate them, as we would have done once upon a time. All of which has the potential to influence the quality of our breathing and therefore to affect the balance of our nervous system.

A typical day for most of us might run something like this:

You wake up to the sound of the alarm on your phone; you pick it up and switch it off and, before you have a chance to think about how you feel, an alert pops up to remind you of your morning meetings.

You check into your tracker to see how well you slept, and it tells you that you woke up three times in the night, and this makes you feel anxious, as you have a big day ahead and now feel tired. As you walk down the hallway to the bathroom, you check Twitter: you learn about atrocities in a country far away, and see devastating photographs of fire-bombed buildings, strewn clothing, and children's shoes. Your heart is in your throat as you brush your teeth, and you are feeling sad for people you have never met. The sadness makes you feel powerless. You then check in to Instagram and see that someone has left a personal comment about you publicly, for all to see. You are mortified.

You get dressed and at the same time are frantically typing out damage-limitation replies to the comment, which means that you have no time for breakfast and run to catch your bus. The bus is full; you manage to squeeze in next to someone with no self-awareness and they take up more space than anyone else and play inappropriate music, loud enough that you can hear it jangling in your ears: who listens to house music at 8 a.m. in the morning? You imagine all the germs being breathed out by everyone else, and this makes you feel anxious.

You get into work and grab a croissant and a coffee, then walk straight into a meeting. The whole day is rushed and frantic and you have no time to go out for lunch, but instead ask someone to grab you a sandwich, which you wolf down at your desk, with your eyes glued to your screen.

You leave work later than you meant to, then there is admin or chores to do when you get home. Your partner has ordered takeout: who has time to cook during the week these days? You pour a glass of wine: you deserve a treat after another hard day at work, and you eat your meal while you catch up with your family. Getting your children organized and into bed takes the last bit of energy you have.

You need to do a bit more work in the evening to be ready for an early-morning meeting, then decide that you need to watch a bit of mindless TV to help you unwind. Unwittingly you end up in bed past midnight, despite your best intentions. You get to sleep quite quickly but wake up several times during the night and it takes you a while to fall asleep again. When your alarm goes off, you feel shattered and anxious about the day ahead.

Does any or all of this scenario sound familiar to you? When you see someone else's typical day laid out like this, it's clear that there are no rests, no pauses, no time to think, to process, to recalibrate, breathe, or daydream. All these triggers throughout the day have the potential to send your nervous system into overdrive.

Added to this, the signals from your body are alerting your nervous system that your muscles, connective tissue, organs, and bones are taking the strain of sitting down for most of the day. You may also not have slept properly or eaten an array of nutritious fresh food, which your gut and brain require to function well. You may not have been outside in daylight or have allowed your gaze to softly release, surrounded by the soothing colors and shapes in nature. Now you have many factors nudging your nervous system into a sympathetic response, or your "go" mode. If this happens consistently, all your systems are playing catch-up to keep you functioning and, instead of living to your full capacity, you are merely surviving. And it makes you feel miserable, anxious about the future and hopeless.

We need to release our system from the bouts of activity so that our brains aren't always switched to the "go" setting. This approach will build a resilient nervous system that can move us away from danger and then recalibrate, so that we are not fixed in either the "go" or "no-go" state. If your nervous system is stuck in the "go" part, this causes sustained stress, and the long-term effects of chronic stress take their toll on your mental and physical health. Chronic stress contributes to high blood pressure and brain changes that may lead to anxiety, depression, and addiction, as well as sleep issues.[3]

Poor posture and breathing

Throughout this book we will examine all the elements that influence your nervous system. As we are focusing on the breath in this chapter, let's look at how you organize your posture and how this can impact on your breathing.

When you are in the same position for long periods of time you run the risk of putting pressure on your internal organs, including your lungs. The lungs should have an elastic, springy quality to them, but long periods of inertia prevent them from inflating fully, as the forces of gravity pull your head, shoulders, and upper spine downward. Your chest muscles tighten and pull you into a forward-folding position, which weakens the back muscles and impacts on your lungs. This means that you may not be breathing to the full capacity of your lungs and, when this happens, your breath becomes shorter and you need to take more breaths per minute in an attempt to get more oxygen into your system.

Unwittingly, in a poorly organized posture you keep some muscles in a contracted state and others in a stretched state to accommodate this held position. Your diaphragm doesn't now fully contract downward or recoil effortlessly, because your front ribs sink and inhibit the movement of the muscles and connective tissues between the bones. Your heart must work harder because of your collapsed posture.

Your energy has now shifted to compensating for the

extra work in keeping you functioning, and this takes energy away from other functions—energy that could be used for digesting, restoring, recalibrating, and repairing your system to maintain biological fitness. When you are biologically fit, all your systems function at their optimal pace, including your mental and physical fitness and your ability to sleep, repair, reproduce, and adapt to your environment.

Consider how different all this would be in a functionally organized posture that allows your lungs to take up their due space and expand and retract with more ease.

Case study: Maisie

In the fast-paced, always switched-on culture we all live in, you are probably very aware of events happening in your environment and in the wider world, because of the twenty-four-hour news cycle. And with the rise of social media, there is no escape: your downtime may consist of streamed movies or box sets, which means that you consume a lot of events, experiences, feelings, and emotions in short, concentrated bursts. Where once you might have stood in a line allowing yourself to daydream or glaze over, now you are more likely to be using that time to buy a dress, book a restaurant, or plan a vacation.

I have a client named Maisie who lived her life with extreme stimulation all around her. She owned a television that was almost as big as the wall it was mounted upon. Whenever I went to see her, she had a movie on at the loudest volume, and it was always a thriller or murder mystery or something that was emotionally discombobulating. But she wasn't watching it; it was on in the background, taking up the air space. If the telephone rang, she would answer it and have a conversation alongside the TV blaring out, the radio on in another room, and at the same time she'd also try to have a conversation with me. I felt so over-stimulated in the first ten minutes of entering her house that I had to employ all my soothing skills to keep my own nervous system steady.

Maisie was never prepared for our sessions—she was in the middle of many different projects at the same time. As she tidied up her belongings and made space on the floor, she would go off on another tangent, showing me something that she was working on or a new record that she had bought. Maisie was well-off and this gave her access to so many distractions. Bags of unopened shopping from high-end boutiques were piled up in corners; she was often out at the latest restaurant, and the clothes, handbag, and shoes that she had worn the night before were strewn on the banisters or on a chair. She was out every night and went to bed late and woke up late.

She didn't enjoy being at home on her own, and would arrange impromptu gatherings to entice people round to her house. I had to spend the first twenty minutes of our sessions coaxing her to switch off each piece of technology, one by one, before she could settle on the floor in readiness. By the end of the session she was peaceful and calm, but she found the concept of becoming quieter and smaller challenging. She hated silence; she told me it made her think. And when Maisie thought about things, she would be overwhelmed with emotions she did not want to feel.

Maisie had had a difficult childhood and had been in therapy for decades. And while therapy had been useful in engaging her cognitive mind—the adult, rationalizing part of her—to help her make sense of her upbringing, the other parts of her that had responded to this at the time had become locked in a protective physical state that kept her stuck in the same patterns of anxiety.

If you remember from Chapter 2 on the senses, your physical body influences your thoughts and emotions. Childhood traumas happen at a time when you have no language for what you go through, so you respond in and with your body. Babies and infants experience the world through their whole self, their mind, their body, and their sensations: they don't differentiate between these parts of themselves. When something happens to you when you are young, you experience and store it, with and in your whole self. When you don't involve your whole self in healing, your experience becomes stuck in your body and inhibits how you respond.

This concept is the work of the psychiatrist and bestselling trauma author Bessel van der Kolk; in his seminal book *The Body Keeps the Score* he explores the question of how we can help people to live in their bodies in a way that makes them feel safe. He posits that good psychotherapy works to help understand and contextualize events, and validates their responses, and that this acknowledgment is an important part of healing from trauma. Your feelings emanate from your body. To heal and move on from that which happens to you, you need to have a deep relationship with your internal sensory system. This idea has been updated by the neuroscientist Lisa Feldman Barrett, who suggests that in fact it is *your brain that keeps the score, while your body is the scorecard.*

I've found that many people don't like to have the space to think, because they then realize that the world is more complicated than the simplistic idea we are sold: the idea that you can think yourself happy by always being positive. That filling your life with noise, products, and experiences can somehow push out the unpleasant stuff you feel, even though distracting attention from how you feel does not resolve this.

Maisie had no awareness of her pattern of breathing: her breath was shallow and in her chest. She took many breaths in and fewer breaths out, as though she was filling up on life. Once she got the hang of a more regular breath pattern, she was able to breathe lower into her lungs. From this, she could release the muscles associated with her breathing so that the process of breathing became effortless. I showed her how she could use this awareness to divert her thoughts, to keep bringing her back to a calm and regular breathing pattern and to notice where she felt her body tense when she had uncomfortable thoughts. Maisie felt she was often teetering on the brink of an anxiety attack, but by calming down her breath she became attuned to experiencing more nuanced feelings.

Slowly, over time, Maisie was able to notice uncomfortable physical sensations or an uncomfortable thought and release them with the breath and with small movements, so that they could be discharged from her system.

A 2009 study concluded that your brain processes about 70,000 thoughts per day,[4] and consumes the equivalent of around 34 gigabytes of information each day,[5] including words, images, radio, TV, video, and advertisements. As smartphones became widely available from 2007 onward, it would be reasonable to assume that this figure is now many times higher.

This never-ending source of information is highly stimulating for your nervous system and will have an influence on how you breathe, how much of your lungs you breathe into and how efficiently you are getting oxygen into your cells. To discern what is causing you emotional distress, you need to pause long enough to investigate what is creating the discomfort. Are you worried about something that is happening right now? In which case remove yourself from the situation causing you the distress. Or is it that you are exhausted and your tired brain quickly responds in a way that is familiar because it saves time? What if, instead of reacting immediately, you pause and give yourself time to get curious about your emotion?

We need to find better descriptions for how we feel

Our emotions are complex and nuanced, and often no single word can accurately describe them. This can make it difficult to communicate to others *how* we feel and can make it hard to understand and regulate our emotions.

Using vague or inaccurate language to describe our emotions can send mixed signals to our nervous system. This can lead to confusion and dysregulation, manifesting as physical symptoms such as anxiety, headaches, or stomachaches. Whenever someone tells me they are "fine," I picture the words *"F***ing Insane, Neurotic, Exhausted"* floating above their heads like a thought bubble.

If you say that you are "stressed" but you don't really know what that means, your nervous system may interpret this as a threat. This can trigger responses, leading to a range of physical and emotional symptoms. On the other hand, finding more precise language to describe your emotions, and relating them to a physical sensation, can help your nervous system understand what is happening and respond accordingly. For instance, if you say that you are feeling "anxious about a presentation" you have to give, and you sense that you are "breathing fast into the upper chest," then you can breathe more slowly, direct your breath lower, into your belly, and shift the focus for your nervous system to deal with the specific task at hand and thus avoid becoming trapped in an alarmed state.

I use movement to help with emotional regulation, by providing a safe and supportive space for people to explore their emotions. In a Soothe session, you are guided through a series of exploratory movements that bring awareness to your body. This is useful to identify the areas that you tense and hold whenever you experience a specific emotion. This improves the connection between the brain and the body and can be used to help people become more aware of their emotions and find better ways to express them.

Paying attention to how you move sends signals to your nervous system that you are safe and relaxed. This can help to reduce the activation of the "go" part of your nervous system and activate the "no-go" part, to promote a state of calm and well-being.

One study found that people who could describe their emotions in detail could better regulate them and cope with stress. This suggests that more granular descriptions of our emotions can help us better understand and manage them.[6]

Conscious breathing at times of difficulty will enable you to calmly assess what you are experiencing in the moment. The first step to change how you do things is to notice where you are right now. When you do this, you will understand how your physical state, alongside the intensity of stimulation in your environment, can make your breathing less efficient. There is a suggestion that health problems such as Alzheimer's, heart disease,[7] diabetes,[8] and sleep issues could in part be caused by not breathing properly.

A new study has found that breathwork may reduce the risk of Alzheimer's disease.[9] The study showed that adults, both old and young, who practiced slow breathing for twenty minutes twice a day for four weeks had lower levels of the proteins thought to contribute to Alzheimer's disease. The study's authors say that the findings suggest that breathwork may be a promising new intervention for Alzheimer's-disease prevention. They caution that more research is needed to confirm these findings but say that the results are encouraging.

In addition to promoting relaxation, slow, deep breathing has also been shown to increase melatonin production. Melatonin is an essential sleep-inducing hormone that promotes the "no-go" tone of your nervous system and inhibits your "go" tone. "No-go" tone is associated with relaxation and rest, while "go" tone is associated with alertness and activity.

The production of melatonin is regulated by the body's circadian rhythm, which is a natural twenty-four-hour cycle that controls sleep-wake patterns. When we are exposed to darkness, the body produces more melatonin, which helps us fall asleep. Slow, deep breathing can help to promote darkness-induced melatonin production, which may lead to better sleep quality. In addition to promoting sleep, melatonin also has a number of other health benefits, including: reducing inflammation, boosting the immune system, protecting against cancer and slowing down the aging process.

When you breathe slowly and at a regular pace, you improve brain function via enhanced circulation in the brain, feeding every cell in the body.[10]

Let's now take some time to look at the structures that

allow you to breathe and how they function: the more you can imagine your lungs and the pathway of oxygen coming into and out of the body, the more you will be able to visualize breathing into them.

Your body in breathing

When you breathe in through your nostrils, the air is warmed and filtered as it travels through the back of your throat and into your windpipe. The air then branches out from your windpipe into your two lungs. You have a right lung and a shorter left lung, which has made space to hug around your heart. The air enters your lungs into tubes called bronchi, which branch out into smaller tubes called bronchioles, which in turn branch out into air sacs called alveoli. The structure looks a bit like a tree: imagine that your windpipe is the trunk, which turns into the branches of the bronchi; the twigs are the bronchioles, and the leaves are the alveoli where the exchange of gases happens.

Oxygen is picked up by blood vessels that surround the alveoli, and they drop off carbon dioxide. This exchange of gases is called respiration. The oxygen is taken from the alveoli through blood vessels into the left side of the heart, which pumps it around the body. When the oxygen is used up, the blood travels into the right side of the heart and then back into the lungs to drop off carbon dioxide and pick up more oxygen. Because oxygen is so crucial to staying alive, your brain prioritizes messages from the lungs above all else.

Your heart sits in between your lungs and pumps the blood around your body. Your diaphragm sits underneath your lungs and above your liver on the right and your stomach.

They have an intimate relationship with each other through sliding joints massaged by the rhythm of your breathing. Your posture affects the quality of your breathing.

The importance of posture isn't about how it looks to other people from the outside: think about it more in terms of how your internal systems are organized. Your bones are designed to stack up against gravity; the curves of the spine dissipate the forces of gravity and your organs are suspended. Your head is carried by the structure underneath it; rather than thinking of your body sinking down into the floor, think about using the bones of your feet to support you upward through your bones, skin, connective tissue, and organs, all the way up to the top of your head.

Your ribs are suspended from your neck by three thick neck muscles, which attach to your first two ribs all the way down to your sixth rib. These muscles are multidirectional in their structure, and the fascia (remember the sashimi in plastic wrap?) that covers them creates the ability for movement in all directions. This structure is echoed in the muscles between the ribs, called the intercostals, as well as in the deep abdominals. The twelfth rib is anchored to the pelvis by another set of three muscles in your lower back. Think of your ribs as being more like a hanging basket than a cage. Imagine the movement of a vertical accordion: as you breathe in, the accordion pulls apart upward and downward; as you breathe out, the accordion pushes the air out by drawing back in.

All these structures are influenced by their common attachments to your breathing body. If the body is static for long periods of time, this has an influence beyond muscles and bone, your internal rhythms are also affected by not moving and by using your energy to stay in a fixed position.

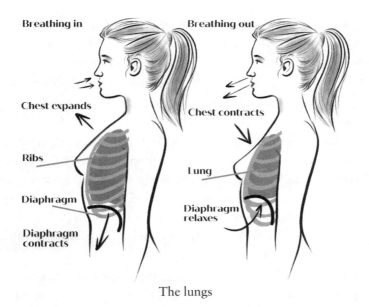

The lungs

As you inhale, the first and second ribs draw up and away from the pelvis as the neck muscles shorten; the muscles in the back of the torso hold the last rib down to increase the length and depth of your ribs and to increase the volume of the lungs to allow for the air to come in. As the diaphragm pulls down, it also pulls the lungs down to take in air. As you exhale, the diaphragm recoils back up and the air is pushed out of the lungs. This multi-ply organization gives a spring-like quality to the ribs, which enables you to increase the length of the rib structure on every inhale.

You also have fascial linings that travel on the front and back of the ribs, and these are continuous with your neck muscles and your lower-back muscles—this gives an idea of you as a continuous elastic structure.

Your lungs are spongy forms encased in a lining that folds back on itself to form a two-layer sac. The outer layer attaches to the chest wall and the inner layer covers the lungs, nerves, blood vessels, and bronchi. The opening up of the ribs enables these linings to slide against each other and open the lungs.

The lungs hang from the collarbone to the eighth rib at the front, and lower down to the tenth rib at the back. However, the linings of the lungs sit above the first rib, so you could say that the lungs hang from the neck. The *lining of the lungs* is attached to the inside of the neck muscles. How you position your head and your neck will hugely influence what happens in respiration.

Your neck is a junction for many important structures that travel into the upper body. The nerves that feed your head, face, and eyes emanate from the back of your neck. You have an important nerve on each side of the neck called the phrenic nerve, which is the only one in the nervous system responsible for movement of the diaphragm. When this nerve fires, your diaphragm contracts, and when it stops firing, your diaphragm expands.

Your phrenic nerve starts at the part of your neck that you use to bend or rotate your head; the part that is level with your jaw. It travels through to your neck, chest, and past your heart and lungs, into your diaphragm. The phrenic nerve also sends sensory information to do with touch and pain to your diaphragm, to the sac covering your heart, to the thin tissue covering your abdominal organs and to the outer lung lining.

There are twelve pairs of cranial nerves that emerge from the brain stem at the back of the skull. These nerves control a variety of functions, including vision, hearing, taste, smell, touch, movement, and balance; they also control messages from your body to your brain and back again. They relate to the movement and sensation of your head, face, neck, shoulders, arms, hands, and fingers. Your neck is also the junction for many muscles that attach to your collarbones, breastbone, the muscles responsible for your shoulder blades, and the skull.

All of this serves to emphasize how influential posture is on your breathing. Any disorganization in any part of the structure lower down, or above, will influence how well you stack up against gravity to allow space in your internal body, so that you use your lungs to their maximum capacity.

Remember the body-mapping that we looked at in Chapter 1? If you are not fully breathing into your lungs because you are habitually hunched forward over your laptop, then you are unwittingly shaping your body map to take up less space in your brain's image of you. This means that you are not using your lungs to full capacity. This signals to the brain that you are stressed, and for the appropriate cascade of responses to activate. If you repeat this, day in and day out, you adapt to this posture and to shorter breath, and your nervous system adapts to this version of you.

Rather than feeling overwhelmed with this information, or even deflated because you sit at a desk all day, know that you are in control of improving this idea of yourself—your self-image—by increasing awareness of your whole self, just as you did when you were a baby. All it needs to kick-start the process of awareness is your attention.

Awareness of your lungs

Let's try a breathing lesson to improve your awareness of your lungs.

1 Either lie down with your knees bent and your feet on the floor or, if you prefer, sit up on your sit bones with your feet on the floor.

2 Lightly place your hands on your mid-ribs just underneath your chest or bust, with your last fingers roughly in line with the bottom of your breastbone before the ribs part away. This is where the lower lobes of your lungs reside. Tune in to the warmth of the palms on your ribs. Breathe into your hands.

3 As you inhale through your nose, breathe into your lungs and feel them expand into your ribs and then into your hands. As you exhale, imagine your ribs and then your lungs retracting away from your hands.

4 Practice this in such a way that you are not using a hard push-pull action with your muscles; make it softer than that—imagine that your hands and lungs are responding to each other under the layers of skin, connective tissue, fluids, elastic lungs, and bone.

5 Continue breathing, but let your hands come down by your sides. Can you still feel the warmth of your hands? You are now aware of your lower ribs and are most likely breathing lower into your ribs. You have just changed the mapping of your lungs in your brain and, with that, you have altered the way you breathe.

Nasal breathing versus mouth breathing

There has been much research on the benefits of breathing through your nose as opposed to breathing through your mouth.

The benefits are that the nose is the first line of defense for the body, by filtering the incoming air. It humidifies, moistens and warms the inhaled air, allowing you to extract 20 percent more oxygen, due to the constriction of breathing in through your nose, the pressure buildup and the resultant release of nitric oxide. Nitric oxide relaxes the inner muscles of the blood vessels, causing them to widen and increase circulation; it is antiviral, antibacterial, and antimicrobial.

Nasal breathing will slow down your breathing, improve your lung capacity and strengthen your diaphragm. It aids your immune system and lowers the likelihood of snoring. Breathing through your mouth increases the risk of asthma, exposure to allergens, bad breath, tooth decay, gum inflammation, dry mouth, and snoring or sleep apnea.[11]

The more you use the full capacity of your lungs, the better they will function and the longer you will live. Your lungs shrink as you get older, but you can change this with your physical posture and by nasal breathing at a slower pace to retain your lung capacity.

How you breathe affects every system of your body: how your brain functions; the pace of your heart; your circulation; your digestion. Slow breathing helps your digestion in a few ways. First, it helps to relax the body and mind. When you are relaxed, your digestive system can function more effectively. When you are stressed, your body releases hormones that can slow down digestion. Slow breathing can also help to increase the production of digestive enzymes, which are essential for breaking down food and absorbing nutrients. It also helps to improve circulation, increasing blood flow to the digestive system. This is important for delivering nutrients to the intestines and for removing waste products by improving liver function. Slow breathing can also assist in reducing pain associated with digestive problems such as indigestion, gas, and bloating.

The 6:6 breath lesson

This type of breathing is also known as coherent breath or resonant breath, although "6:6 breath" most clearly describes what it is.

1   Either lie down with your knees bent or sit up on your sit bones with your feet on the floor.
2   Place one hand on your belly, then let your elbow drop down.
3   Breathe in through your nose for a slow count of six and let your belly rise.
4   Breathe out through your nose for a slow count of six and let your belly fall.
5   Once you get used to the pace of breathing you can start restricting the back of the throat lightly, so that your breath sounds like a baby snoring. Try not to over-restrict the back of the throat; this is soft and should not take too much effort.

You may find one part of this breathing more challenging than the other. When I first started to practice this pace of breath many years ago I had difficulty exhaling to this count.

But the more I allowed my breath to feel like a continuous loop, where the inhale transitions smoothly into the exhale, the more my muscles relaxed into it.

If you find it challenging, you can always start with three seconds and slowly build up to six, but I've found that most of the people I teach can usually drop into it with regular practice.

Slow and lower breathing

This pace of breathing will slow you down to five breaths per minute, which is made up of: 1 breath = 12 seconds (six seconds inhale, six seconds exhale) × 5 breaths = 1 minute.

Studies show that breathing at a pace of around five to seven breaths per minute can balance, strengthen, and create resilience in our stress response systems, counteracting the effects of excess stress and trauma on our emotion-regulation and physical health.[12] Breathing at this pace allows the nervous system to swing between the sympathetic ("go") and parasympathetic ("no-go") response with each inhalation and exhalation, which results in balance. This is because the inhalation is enlivening and activates the "go" part of your nervous system, whereas the exhalation activates the "no-go" response.

This breathing pace existed in ancient practices. The religious chants "Ave Maria" and "OM" are at five breaths per minute, when practiced. Science has verified something that has been around for a long time.

From the work of breath and science practitioners Dr. Richard Brown and Dr. Patricia Gerberg, we know that breathing and emotion are neurologically connected.[13] Your body continuously relays information to your brain, keeping it updated on the internal state of your body. This intricate communication network is crucial for maintaining your well-being. From the sensory receptors throughout your body to the delicate sensors lining your lungs and airways, a constant stream of data flows to your brain. This information, updated in milliseconds, ensures that your brain remains informed about your breathing, a vital process that delivers life-sustaining oxygen.

When you change the pattern of your breathing, you are changing the pattern of the signals that are going to the brain: certain breathing patterns signal that you are in danger and others signal that you are safe. Specific emotions elicit distinct breathing patterns. For instance, feeling startled can induce a holding of breath, a response that further reinforces the emotional state through the corresponding breathing pattern.

By consciously changing your breathing you alter the patterns of the respiratory signals that go to the lower part of your brain, which is connected to your spinal cord— *the brain stem*—and from this to all the major regulatory networks in the brain: the emotion centers, the internal communication systems, the thinking and decision-making centers, and many aspects of emotional and cognitive processes. If you can pause to work out what breathing pattern you need to bring you back to a state of calm, you will have an impact upon the entire function of the brain.

You can affect the rate you breathe at by the relationship between the inhale and the exhale, and by the different lengths of breath. You can breathe gently or with force, or create resistance in the breath, such as when you restrict the back of the throat. The easiest way to affect the "no-go" part of your nervous system is by slowing down to five breaths per minute.

The benefits of this pace of breathing have been shown for individuals with psychiatric and medical conditions, at-risk children, veterans, and survivors of disasters.[14]

How to practice

Consistency is important, and regular practice when your mind is calm and quiet first thing in the morning works well, because your brain hasn't been scrambled by your day. Twenty minutes of slow breathing per day has been shown to be optimal to balance your nervous system, but you can start with two minutes per day, build up to five minutes and slowly upward from there.

A powerful way to create a new habit is to attach it to an old one, so as soon as I wake up, I sit up in bed and practice this slow breathing for twenty minutes and then I am ready for my day. If, for any reason, I don't manage to fit it in, I'll do it at another point in my day. I also use it throughout the day whenever I need it to recover and reset my nervous system.

I will share many practices in this book, but the 6:6 breath is the foundation for bringing your nervous system into balance. Make it your go-to daily practice—try it consistently for a month and see what changes you notice.

Breathing to soothe digestive issues

If you are experiencing digestive problems, slow breathing can be a helpful way to improve your symptoms. You can try practicing slow breathing for ten to fifteen minutes a day or whenever you feel your digestion is off. Here are some simple steps on how to do it:

1   Sit in a comfortable position, with your spine long.
2   Close your eyes and focus on your breath.
3   Breathe in slowly through your nose for a count of four.
4   Hold your breath lightly for a count of four.
5   Breathe out slowly through your mouth for a count of four.
6   Repeat steps 3–5 for ten to fifteen minutes.

What you have learned in this chapter

- Your breath controls your nervous system, so if you breathe in a dysfunctional way, you put all these systems of your body in a state of stress.
- Your emotions and your breathing are intimately connected neurologically.
- A slow and steady 6:6 pace of breath is the easiest way to calm your nervous system as it creates balance between the "go" and "no-go" parts of your nervous system.
- The position of your head, neck, and spine will affect the signals from your body to your brain.
- Your physical state affects your ability to breathe to your full capacity.
- When you breathe low into your lungs, it activates the "no-go" part of your nervous system: rest, repair, and digest; reproduce and restore.

- The inhale stimulates the "go" part of your nervous system, while the exhale balances it by activating the "no-go" part.

Take a slow breath in through your nose and a slow breath out, and perhaps take a break, go outside and let your brain rest. Breathing outside in nature with soft eyes is the perfect way to let this information marinate in your brain.

In the next chapter we will move on to learning about the importance and significance of *touch*.

4

Touch

The skin is our largest organ, and it is through
touch that we experience the world around us.

Ashley Montagu, *Touching: Human Significance of the Skin*

What is the first thing you think about when you read the word "touch"? Do you conjure up feeling safe and loved? Or does the word make you feel vulnerable and fearful? Perhaps you immediately think about sexual or sensual touch, or massage or therapeutic touch. Your experience of touch will shape your worldview.

Case study: Alistair

I have a client—let's call him Alistair—who feels so bereft of love that he buys as much touch-time as he can with frequent massages, manicures, pedicures, and even facials. He says that it makes him feel loved. He told me that his mother did not kiss or cuddle him. She had been sent to London from Poland, aged eleven in 1923, by the authorities with a letter containing her particulars and asking anyone who encountered her on the journey to kindly help her. She was met at Victoria station by a distant relative living in the East End of London, who was to look after her. Her mother (Alistair's grandmother) had died in childbirth and her father (his grandfather) had been hanged from a lamp post by an anti-Semitic mob. His mother had been so traumatized by this experience that when she became a mother, she couldn't hug or kiss her children.

Alistair does not know how to self-regulate his emotions. When he gets upset, he doesn't understand how to soothe his system to feel calmer. His emotions often overwhelm him and, when this happens, he either goes to sleep or engages in disruptive behavior to numb his feelings. Alistair is drawn to action: he enjoys days when he is fully scheduled, down to the last minute. He will do anything to fill in space and any quiet time, to ensure that he doesn't have time to think or to *feel* his feelings.

When I first started to teach Alistair, whenever I asked him to get on the floor at the start of our sessions, it wouldn't be very long before he fell asleep. He didn't understand that filling every moment in the day and repeating this until bedtime is exhausting. He was either in "on" mode or "off" mode. He didn't sleep well at night; he would breathe predominantly through his mouth and he suffered from sleep apnea—this is where your breathing stops and starts in your sleep, you make gasping or choking noises and it wakes you up throughout the night; it is commonly associated with snoring. The next day sufferers feel very tired, find it hard to focus, and experience mood swings because they haven't completed their sleep cycles. (I will talk more about sleep cycles in Chapter 6.) Sometimes people with sleep apnea may also suffer from headaches. Alistair had all these symptoms. He was continually exhausted and would regularly drink eight to ten big cups of coffee a day to stay awake.

He was overweight and uncomfortably so, had gout and took pills for blood pressure, high cholesterol, and diabetes. His approach to life was that if it felt good, he wanted more of it: more food, more experiences, and more people around him. He loved collecting things. He had containers of antiques that he bought in auctions, but they went straight into storage. If he loved something, he wanted to repeat it again and again—be it his favorite TV show, a film, or an enjoyable meal. He had a long marriage, but not a happy one, and felt lonely and unloved.

Alistair is also one of the most successful people I know. It is almost as if his lack of self-awareness has allowed him to be utterly fearless in business and not think of the consequences of his actions. There is something about him that gives him a lack of awareness; he has displayed neurodiverse tendencies, but has never been diagnosed, nor would he want to be. It is not my job to diagnose, and it is better that I don't know what labels have been attached to a client. They don't have to tell me anything about their "story." Instead I guide them through movements, and I observe where they are holding themselves stuck in a pattern that stops them breathing fully or moving with ease. We work together very gently to help unlock that pattern.

I showed Alistair how to move when he senses that his feelings have welled up inside him; and how to soothe himself using breath, touch, and movement practices, which he can now do and he understands how to manage his feelings. He resonated with any lesson where he had to use touch, as this helped him to understand his relationship to himself and his environment. For instance, if I asked him to roll up from a forward fold into a standing pose, no matter how many times I emphasized the words "slowly" or "gently" or "your head comes up last," Alistair would unroll as quickly as possible and experience a head rush. But when I asked him to place his hands on the top of his feet and slide his hands up his shins, thighs, pelvis, belly, and chest to unroll into a standing pose, and finally bring his head up last, it worked for him. He had to feel the unrolling of his body with his hands in order to comprehend how he moved his body in space.

In most of his sessions I would guide him to feel the movement of his breath on his rib basket, with his hands, and this is how he came to understand 6:6 breathing (see page 100) and could practice it for a length of time; or I would get him to use props so that he had feedback to sense himself against the boundaries of the prop. Getting Alistair to use all of his senses was most useful in getting him to *feel*.

He has lost fifty-six pounds and has finally thrown away his bigger-sized clothes, which he kept over the decades in case he put the weight back on. He is now better at breathing through his nose, he sleeps well, his sleep apnea has evaporated, his coffee consumption is down to one cup a day and his gout has completely cleared up.

I sometimes see in Alistair the young child who craved touch and, because he didn't get it, found ways to soothe himself with so many other distractions.

In contrast to Alistair, another client (let's call her Lucy) cannot bear to be touched unexpectedly, as it makes her freeze. She had grown up in a household where both her parents were long-term substance abusers. Their behavior was erratic and unpredictable, and they struggled to recognize their own needs as well as those of their young child. This made Lucy hypervigilant. My work is mainly online, but sometimes I see clients in person, as there is a hands-on element to my work, which is useful for those clients who have little awareness of their own sensations. I always make sure that I announce what I am going to be doing in advance of putting my hands on in-person clients, but I must be particularly aware of giving Lucy advance notice and must ask her permission. I also give her many options to settle herself, so that she can choose whether she wants her eyes open or not. The Soothe Program is well suited to her because it gives her agency over her own body and comfort. We have worked together to calm her nervous system, so that touching someone or being touched doesn't send her into a complete panic.

How do we learn how to care for ourselves? According to trauma experts, you learn how to care for yourself from the way your caregiver cared for you. Did they soothe you when you were upset? Did they scold, shake, hit, or ignore you?

The importance of touch in early life experience plays a fundamental role in how the social brain forms. I clearly remember seeing the haunted faces of Romanian orphans on television when the outside world first discovered news of the state orphanages in the 1990s. Those infants were the result of a brutal regime presided over by the dictator Nicolae Ceaușescu; he had decided that Romania needed to expand its population to become a more profitable nation. Birth control and abortion were banned, and childless people were heavily taxed. When parents could not cope with the financial and emotional burdens of additional children, especially if they were physically disabled, they were sent to state orphanages. Aside from being fed and changed, the babies were left to fend for themselves in their cots, with no human contact. Knowing that no one would come and comfort them if they cried, they stopped making the sounds of babies who know someone will respond. The news reports showed eerie scenes of silent and feral children looking at the camera, unsmiling. There was no one to comfort them or sing to them or cuddle them, no skin-on-skin touch. They looked like ghost children. It was heartbreaking.

The problems that stem even from less extreme infant neglect include poor emotional regulation, social withdrawal, low self-esteem, delays in motor development and language, poor intellectual functioning, self-harm, and tantrums, and in time this can lead to low academic achievement. Such children suffer from cognitive deficits that last throughout their lives, particularly if they were institutionalized from birth.

Babies learn by exploring their environment, being encouraged, being made to feel safe and trying new things and learning from their mistakes. The brain is made up of different areas that are involved in everything you do, and each area has millions of neurons or brain cells. The neurons involved in these actions communicate with each other by passing chemical messages between them. By repeating an action over and over, the messages between the two neurons will link to form new neural pathways. This process of your brain to change, and to adapt by building new networks, is called neuroplasticity. Babies learn from their environment and their relationships. Neural pathways thrive in babies who are loved, touched, played with, encouraged, and taken care of, because social connection is how they learn and form experiences. You cry and are soothed by your caregiver, which teaches you how to soothe yourself. Your caregiver smiles and coos at you and you learn to smile or gurgle back— this teaches you how to form social relationships.

Nurturing interaction with your caregiver helps to regulate your neurophysiology and includes critical learning,
such as regulating your body; regulating attuned communication with others; emotional balance and empathy; and
modulation of fear.[1] Seeking comfort from a caregiver is
a learned behavior, but those Romanian children didn't
know how to do that because they had never been shown
and had no idea that they could be comforted.

The skin that you are in

Take your palms and rub them together. Can you feel that
there is a thickness to the skin on your palms? Can you feel
the tiny grooves and creases in each hand? Now take a finger
lightly around the underneath of your eye and feel how thin
this skin is. Your skin is versatile and has different qualities,
depending on where it is and what it needs to cover. It will
show the world your experiences of life, as well as the state
of your internal body.

If you think back to Chapter 1, your skin—in common
with your nervous system—is formed by the outer layer of
tissue in the embryo. Also arising from this layer are your
teeth, your hair, and the organs that give you smell, vision,
hearing and taste. Your skin travels inward to form the
insides for your eyelids, ears, nostrils, genitalia, anus, and
mouth: you could think of this as an internal lining of your
skin. Your skin can be considered your external nervous
system; at the same time, your nervous system can be considered your internal "skin," acting as a conduit between
your internal and external environments. Your skin has been
described as the first medium of communication.[2]

As a baby, it's likely you would have used your hands and mouth to find your mother's breast. Your skin, acting as an organ of balance, gives you the information to understand which way you are oriented in space and to receive feedback from your mother stroking and caressing you to further stimulate your brain. Your skin gives you a sense of self that is separate from the skin of the person you embrace—it gives you your boundary.

Your skin has millions of sensory receptors that can receive the different stimuli of heat, cold, pain, pressure, and touch. The tactile sense is the first to form in embryonic development, and your brain gives a sizable part of its real estate to your sensory receptors, which gives you an idea of the importance of your tactile functions.

Touch has been categorized into two different types: the *fast-touch nerve system*, which enables you to detect a mosquito landing on your arm or the heat of a hot pan, and the *slow-touch nerve system*, which enables you to detect a specific kind of slow contact, such as a stroke or a cuddle.[3] The slow-touch nerve system is only present on parts of your body that are covered in hair, such as your forearm, and is not present on the soles of the feet or the palms of your hands. We are wired to connect and bond with others, to reassure, to nurture, to empathize and to understand our sense of *self* and sense of support from others, and the slow-touch nerve system is designed to facilitate this.

Fast touch leads you outward—think about your hands reaching out to experience the world, or your lips or feet in contact with or exploring the external world. Slow touch is more about the internal experience of being human: it helps to regulate your emotions and to develop your social brain.[4]

Touch has a fundamental influence on how we function. We now know that babies who are premature need to be touched in incubators to allow for the social bonding that happens between mother and child. The development of the social brain requires touch; it is necessary for healthy cognitive, social, emotional, and physical development.

Over the course of writing this book, a litter of puppies arrived accidentally in our household, and the mother dog, who was still quite young herself, knew instinctively to lick her offspring. Licking is essentially touch and is vital for dogs, particularly around the perineum, that space between their genitals and anus. If this doesn't take place, the puppy is unlikely to survive, due to failure of the reproductive, urinary and digestive systems.[5]

Owning a dog can bring about a fast track to familiarity, simply because you spend time walking the same circuit around a park and gathering with other dog owners at specific spots. I remember a woman I met in the park on my dog walks. One day she tearfully confided in me that her husband had recently left her. She was naturally upset about it, and I wanted to hug her to show empathy and support. However, we were in the first lockdown of the pandemic, I didn't know her and she didn't know me, so neither of us felt we could do that. Not only were the rules strict concerning contact with people outside your immediate circle, but everyone was quite anxious about their own health and about encroaching on other people's personal space. In that moment I experienced two conflicting experiences at the same time, cognitively understanding one thing, but *feeling* another—this is known as "cognitive dissonance." I remember it as an extremely unfulfilling interaction, which still unsettles me whenever I think about it. The urge to comfort others is a strong biological pull and when we resist it, it takes away something from us as well in some way.

Hugging has been shown to have a calming influence on both the hugger and the huggee. The extended bodily contact stimulates the nervous system, and the brain's emotional processing networks get activated, producing neurochemicals including *oxytocin*. This is known as the "cuddle hormone" as it serves to make you feel good, foster social bonding and reduce stress and anxiety levels. It also helps fight off infection and slow down your heart rate. Regular hugging can reduce your reactivity to stress and build your resilience. If you share a bed with someone, gentle touch will help to regulate your sleep by lowering your levels of cortisol, the "go" hormone.[6]

The more you touch and hug your partner or children, the more you create a positive feedback loop and increase each other's oxytocin levels. In one study, researchers found that twenty seconds of hugging a partner decreased their stress levels before the potentially demanding event of public speaking.[7]

You can also increase your own and your pet's oxytocin levels by regular stroking—but if you have a pet, you already know that. I often think I should pay my dogs for their therapeutic service.

Touch is quite a touchy subject (!). There are codes around touch in education and public spaces, and we do need safeguards in society to ensure that boundaries of trust are not broken. However, touch is an immediate way to relax the nervous system and it would be a shame to feel wary about touching ourselves without it having a sexual connotation—

or to avoid touching other people platonically, especially people that we know.

Use touch to soothe

I enjoy the daily ritual of massaging my face every morning. I started during the pandemic, when there was no professional means of looking after myself. It made me realize how important going to the hairdresser's for a blow-dry or having my nails done was to me. I've kept up facial massage ever since, because the simple action of stroking and smoothing my face feels incredibly soothing on all fronts. Not only does my skin benefit from the increased circulation, but there is something about looking at yourself in the mirror and caring for the part of you that faces outward to the world that feels deeply nurturing. The relationship of my hands to my face feels intuitive, following and accentuating the contours of the bones of my face, jawline, cheekbones, and the bones around the eyes. I use upward movements to reverse the effects of gravity on my face.

Stroking, massaging, and touch not only have an influence on the skin, connective tissue, and muscle, but also help your fluid system to flow. Your lymphatic system acts as a drainage system, moving fluid from your body into your blood. It contains white blood cells that fight infection and gets rid of waste that your cells make, so it is good to get this flowing. Lymph needs muscle action to help it to journey through the system, so light manipulation and movement help this system to function well.

Face-massage lesson

Try this massage to experience the benefits of soothing touch.

1　Rub your palms together with your favorite facial oil. I apply it by pressing it into my face and down to my chest.

2　With your right open hand, stroke upward from your chin to your left ear and down the left side of your neck to help your lymph flow drain downward. Do this three times on each side.

3　Now take your three middle fingers to either side of the base of your neck, just above your collarbones; your fingers should point up in the direction of your head. Lightly pump your fingers here three times.

4　Make fists and take each thumb underneath your jawline on either side of your chin. Stroke the thumbs along the jawline to your ears as you massage your cheeks with your knuckles all the way up to your ears. You can be firm, with your thumb against the index finger pinching the jawline and smoothing the skin up to my ears. Then start again at the chin.

5　Now use your knuckles to draw underneath your cheekbones from the corner of your nose to your ears, as if you are molding cheekbones from clay. Repeat this a few times.

6　Hold your knuckles up underneath your cheekbones and keep them there for a few breaths.

7　Open up your hands and use your middle fingers to stroke upward through the midline of your face, from your chin to the corners of your mouth, the creases around your nose, up between your eyebrows to your hairline.

8 Use your first two fingers and rub them upward from the outer side of one eyebrow across the middle of your forehead to the outer eyebrow on the other side and then up to your hairline. The action involves rubbing one set of fingers upward and then the next set of fingers upward from the opposite side, as if you are going in a zigzag pattern, and doing this at pace so that the skin feels stimulated.

9 Use this rubbing method, but turn your fingers parallel to your eyebrows and slide the left fingers to the right and back again, and the right fingers to the left and back again, as if you are rubbing cream into your forehead.

10 Alternate your hands stroking your forehead: using your right hand, stroke it across your forehead from left to right, and using your left hand from right to left.

11 Take your first two fingers and smooth the skin on top of the bone socket under the eye upward to the temples, then repeat this three times. Now use the same fingers to smooth the skin from the upper brow out to the temples.

12 Next, smooth out the skin with your hands from your nose outward to your hairline.

13 Last of all, repeat step 2, smoothing from your chin to the ear and down the neck, three times on each side.

Getting into the habit of touching your skin compassion-
ately is a deeply nurturing practice and these are just some
ideas for you. Use your hands intuitively on your face so that
you give yourself what you need.

Self-hug lesson

1 Sit on a chair, or you could lie down with your knees
   bent and let your bones drop down to the floor.
2 Notice how you feel and what parts of yourself you
   are aware of. If you are sitting down, you might be
   aware of your sit bones and of your feet on the floor.
   If you are lying down, the back of your head and
   your shoulders might be more apparent to you. Or
   perhaps your shoulders are feeling tight and tense
   from your day?
3 Start to notice your breath: notice how it travels in
   and out through the nostrils. As you inhale, notice
   how your belly rises; and as you exhale, notice how
   your belly falls. Tune in to the expansion on the
   inhale and the retraction on the exhale.
4 Now take your hands and give yourself a hug. You
   are crossing your arms over your chest: you should
   have your right hand on your left arm, and your left
   hand on your right arm. Stroke your hands down
   your arms on your exhale, take your hands off and
   place them back on the tops of your arms, then
   stroke your hands down your arms again. Do this
   a few times, tenderly and softly. Remember to cross
   your arms over in the other direction and start again.
   If you can't get your arms across your chest, you

can stroke down your front from your collarbones
to your lower belly. Allow the strokes to be long and
luxurious. Think about your slow-touch system—
you don't want to rush them.

5 Do this until you feel calmer and able to carry on
with your day. I use this lesson throughout my day
whenever I want to check in with myself or let go of
the work I have been doing.

What you have learned in this chapter

- Slow-touch interactions with other people, such as
  hugs, strokes of the back, and other nonsexual touch
  with friends and family, will soothe your and their
  nervous system.
- Hugging has many benefits, including increasing
  your sense of well-being.
- Your skin is your external nervous system, and
  any irritation of the skin can be traced back to the
  balance of your nervous system. You are a complex
  of interwoven systems that feed into your body's
  master system.

In the next chapter we will look at movement and why it is
about so much more than simply getting your steps in. See
you there.

5

Move

The brain is not just a thinking organ. It is also an organ
of movement. The way we move affects the way we think,
and the way we think affects the way we move. When we
change the way we move, we change the way we think.

Moshé Feldenkrais, *Awareness Through Movement*[1]

We live in a time when our bodies have never been so scru-
tinized and discussed. We are encouraged to push them to
extremes to achieve new personal bests, to beat ourselves in
the gym and to use exercise to sculpt, shape, punish, cajole,
and control. We are bombarded with images of "perfect"—
sometimes surgically enhanced—bodies. From "New Year,
New You" to the "Beach Body," the implicit message is that
what you are in this moment is not good enough. And despite
calls for body positivity, this conditioning means that we're
probably not feeling very positive about our bodies.

Our bodies are an intricate system, and their job is to
maintain homeostasis, or balance, yet we are continually
doing things to disrupt that natural rhythm and seem to
be at constant war with ourselves. We sit down for long
periods, neglect to sleep or rest enough, fill our every waking
moment with some form of activity, pour copious amounts

of caffeine down our throats, and consume foods with myriad ingredients that our poor guts struggle to decipher.

Because we have such a complicated relationship with our bodies, we also feel fraught when it comes to moving them, even though we are designed to move. You might have memories of running around cold, muddy fields at school, along with the humiliation of being the last one chosen for the team. Or are you one of the 80 percent of new gym members who quit after five months of membership? Most people cite the cost of gyms, losing motivation, not seeing results quickly enough and feeling out of place or being too busy as reasons for not exercising. When I ask my clients what stops them moving a little every day, they cite just not feeling motivated enough to do so. Or they have an all-or-nothing approach, where one time they will be intensely engaged in regular fitness classes, but something happens in their life to interrupt that. Their resolve goes out of the window, and they fall into an extended fallow period of not looking after themselves and returning to their habit of long hours of working, little sleep and a lack of nutritious food.

How did it all get so complicated? And how can we cut through this noise and get back to the fundamentals of what matters? I see clients with chronic stress, anxiety, and burnout because they didn't deal with their daily stresses at the time. They stopped prioritizing their care. Now they feel despondent, cynical, exhausted, and emotional. And it's a vicious cycle: the less you move, the less inclined you are to move. My work emphasizes movement to help you self-regulate your emotions, and it has been proven to be effective time and time again. Let's explore why this is.

Why do we move?

Moving through the world and thinking are intimately connected and they evolved when we became hunter-gatherers
and had to forage for food. Our ancestors needed to travel
long distances, and often chased mammals until their prey
was exhausted. In this scenario, you need different skills,
such as thinking and planning where you are going, and
complex thoughts, such as advanced communication skills
and group strategy. You must recognize patterns to follow
animal tracks, and have spatial awareness and navigation
skills. This, combined with the aerobic endurance needed
for the cognitive demands of hunter-gathering, enhances
your neural responses to movement. The human brain's
evolution might be better understood as an adaptation to
movement rather than solely for thinking. Our ancestors'
survival depended on their ability to move, as their food
supply was intimately linked to their physical activity.
Hunter-gatherers covered remarkable distances, traversing
up to fourteen miles daily to secure sustenance. This constant mobility played a crucial role in shaping the human
brain, fostering its development to support movement planning, coordination, and navigation.

Neurotransmitters, or chemical messengers, in the brain
evolved to adapt to long-lasting stressors. Stress causes the
release of chemicals to increase heart rate, slow digestion,
and numb pain, and to release extra glucose in the brain.
This is beneficial in the short term, and because our ancestors were moving on foot for most of their day, they could
self-regulate the release of these chemicals because they were
necessary to keep them moving. The chemicals were released
and metabolized through movement.

Movement is how you experience your environment; your brain has evolved to allow you to do this. You have a brain that enables you to produce adaptable and complex movements. This is the only way you can affect the world around you, and you do this through muscular contractions. If you regularly use a muscle, it will respond to its use by expanding its capacity; if you don't use it, it will shrink its capacity. The brain responds similarly. Physical activity stresses our brains in a good way. Moving through the world is a cognitively demanding task, which enables your brain to stay resilient. In fact the two most expensive things your brain can do, in terms of using up your resources, are to move and to learn something new. But if part of your brain's job is to conserve energy, why move at all?

The answer is that movement in the short term will change your brain chemistry to make you feel more hopeful and energetic. Regular activity over time will actually alter the structure and function of your brain in ways that teach it to be more resilient to stress and more optimistic.

How? When you contract your muscles regularly and continuously, chemicals are released into your bloodstream, reducing inflammation, improving immune and cardiovascular health, and regulating your blood sugar, and even eliminating malformed cells such as cancer cells. Some chemicals released from contracting muscle cross your blood–brain barrier and act as an antidepressant. Your muscles in action deliver these chemicals to your brain to lift your mood.

In a recent study, researchers found that parts of the brain area involved in controlling movement are connected to networks involved in thinking and planning.[2] They also control functions such as blood pressure and heartbeat. This significant finding connects the goal-focused part of your mind to the area of your brain that controls your heart rate and breathing. Breathing is a remote control to dial down an overstimulated brain and nervous system. The findings represent a literal connection of body and mind in the brain's structure.

Modern humans face different kinds of stress, but the biological stress response has stayed the same. Your genes haven't changed much in 10,000 years, but your lifestyle is vastly different. You can order food from the sofa; you don't even have to buy the ingredients and cook them. You spend most of the day sitting, and most of your leisure time watching films, eating, and drinking. You outsource your domestic work, and perhaps you drive to the gym. Your lifestyle has taken out all the potential for movement. You are designed to move, yet your modern lifestyle keeps you still.

What happens when you experience micro-stresses throughout the day without taking any action? The chemicals build up in your body and become inflammation over time. The system designed to save you from stress will slowly kill you if you do not release the stress. There is a differentiation between the events that cause you stress and those that build up as a residue of the stress. Stress is a physical and emotional response to a challenge or threat. It can be caused by anything from a minor annoyance to a major life event. When confronted with a perceived threat or demanding situation, our bodies activate a physiological response known as the fight, freeze, or flight response. This innate survival mechanism, honed over millennia of human evolution, prepares us to respond to danger in one of three fundamental ways: fighting, fleeing, or freezing. Stressors are the events or situations that cause the stress. They can be external, such as a job loss or a car accident, or internal, such as worrying about money or health.

Sustained stress occurs when stress is either prolonged or chronic. This can happen when we are exposed to repeated stressors or when we do not have enough time to recover from stress. Sustained stress can have a negative impact on our physical and mental health.

When we experience stress, our nervous system goes into overdrive. The "go" part of our nervous system is activated, which increases our heart rate, breathing, and blood pressure. This prepares us to fight or flee. The "no-go" nervous system is also activated, but to a lesser extent. This system helps to calm us down and return our bodies to normal.

When stress is prolonged, the sympathetic nervous system, which is responsible for the fight, freeze, or flight response, can become overactive. This can lead to a number of health problems, including:

- heart disease
- high blood pressure
- diabetes
- stroke
- depression
- anxiety
- sleep problems
- weight gain
- memory problems
- gut issues.

I see many clients in my clinic who have these issues. They

often tell me that they feel like they are constantly on edge and can't relax. They may also have trouble connecting with others, feel disengaged, suffer from poor concentration and find it difficult to make decisions.

We have been undersold the importance of movement— or it has been mis-sold to us in a reductive way: to lose weight. Yet movement and being human are intricately intertwined. You reduce your cognitive function when you reduce your movements.

Movement and mood

How does exercise impact on your brain?

You may already be familiar with the euphoria you feel if you've been for a run, a long walk or a cold-water swim. However, there is more to it than just the endorphins that are released during activity. In a study, researchers found that those who exercised for forty-five minutes three to five times a week reported fewer poor mental-health days than those who did not exercise.[3] The study included all types of physical activity, ranging from childcare, housework, lawn-mowing, and fishing, to cycling, going to the gym, running, and skiing.

All types of exercise were associated with lower mental-health burdens. Cycling, aerobics, and going to the gym were associated with the biggest reductions, but team sports seemed to be the activity with a stronger association with good mental health. Social connection helps make you more resilient to stress, so combining movement with other people is an especially effective way to bring about these benefits.

The study showed 40 percent better mental health in people who exercised than in those who did not exercise. The difference in mental health between people who exercised and those who didn't was much more significant than the difference in mental state between people who were obese and those who were healthy.

Movement acts directly on the chemicals that the brain uses to communicate, such as dopamine, which affects mood, motivation, and feelings of well-being and attention. Exercise boosts dopamine and the storage of it. It also boosts serotonin, which modulates mood, impulse control, and self-esteem and helps to keep stress levels in check by counteracting cortisol and enhancing learning.

Exercise regulates a particular molecule in the brain, called brain-derived neurotrophic factor (BDNF for short), keeping neurons healthy, thriving, and communicating faster. BDNF has been shown to enhance mental abilities and act against anxiety and depression in mice, and is thought to act similarly in humans. In a study in the US, a school district improved its students' fitness and academic scores by turning physical education into a more fun, but also more rigorous experience.[4] Students in a remedial literacy program took an extended PE session before classes each day. The district went from lagging behind to outpacing almost all school districts in science and math.

Exercise stimulates the birth of new brain cells, enhancing plasticity and your ability to memorize things is linked to your fitness. Physical activity is also linked to lower levels of inflammation in the blood, which has been shown to help reduce mood disorders. And it improves heart health and controls your emotional and physical stress levels.

Exercise is as good for the mind as it is for the body, with the effect of promoting brain health as we age.[5] Healthy older adults who are physically active are 40 percent less likely than those who are inactive to develop Alzheimer's disease. Physical exercise can also help to slow down the progress of the disease. Aerobic exercise regulates all functions and helps release BDNF to allow faster communication between nerve cells, and to help the brain focus, pay attention, and retain information. It has also been shown to protect against heart and lung disease, cancers, and ADHD, anxiety, addiction, and depression. Parkinson's, dementia, and Alzheimer's are forestalled, alleviated, or even stalled by exercise.

I have firsthand experience of this in my older clients with Parkinson's. If they haven't moved a lot, they appear slow and sluggish, but if they keep up a habit of movement every day, they appear sharper and better able to cope with challenges and exhibit fewer tremors. I have also found that if I can get them to practice their 6:6 breathing (see page 100) as they move, their tremors lessen and their balance improves. Everything works better when the nervous system is in balance. When stressful events and the way you perceive them disrupt your balance, your nervous system will adapt. But it will do so by shutting down functions that are not useful to you for now.

Case study: Ellen

Ellen came to see me because her health was getting steadily worse. She was overweight and had experienced a cascade of health issues over the decades. She suffered from panic attacks, agoraphobia, low moods, asthma, insomnia, high cholesterol, high blood pressure, diabetes, and irritable bowel syndrome. Over the course of our sessions, she told me that both her parents had died in a car crash when she was sixteen and she had to take care of her four younger brothers. She cooked, cleaned, and took them to and from school. She had to ensure they did their homework and kept out of trouble. Her aunt lived a few doors down the road, but the responsibility fell mainly on her.

When she was older, Ellen trained to become a nurse. Being in service to others was her default setting, because she had learned from a young age—and as the only girl in the family—that she had to be the carer. She did not know how to prioritize her own health. Setting a calmer breathing pattern was the first lesson, getting her to notice how she involved her whole body in her breathing. Ellen's body had been such a source of pain and anxiety that she could not feel her physical sensations. Over time she learned to breathe deeper into her lungs, helping her to feel calmer and safer.

I encouraged Ellen to practice breathing in her garden first thing in the morning. This exposed her eyes to daylight, resetting her circadian rhythm. Her breathing practice calmed her mind and empowered her to change her feelings. Over time and with the support of her husband, she scoped out an easy walking route and went for a walk first thing in the morning. She practiced her breathing as she walked. Daily movement lifted her mood and she felt empowered by the corresponding shift of her emotions. She was accustomed to pushing down her feelings. Our sessions explored the habitual movement patterns that influenced her thoughts about her self-worth.

Ellen now has workable strategies to calm her mind, soothe her body and help her back to sleep when she wakes up worrying about her family. She has come off one of her asthma inhalers, has eliminated processed foods from her diet and has learned to roll and jiggle on the floor whenever her feelings overwhelm her. Her lifetime of learned habits and ideas about herself—that life was hard; there was no time for feelings; you had to get on with things; she had to hold everyone together—are slowly being released from her whole self, body and mind.

What is stress?

Stress is an unavoidable part of life. It is the body's natural response to any perceived demand or threat. Stress can manifest in two primary forms: acute stress and chronic stress.

Acute stress is a brief reaction to an abrupt and unanticipated stressor, such as a job interview or a public speaking engagement. During acute stress, the body releases hormones like adrenaline and noradrenaline, which elevate heart rate, breathing rate, and blood pressure. This is the body's mechanism for preparing to fight, freeze, or flee the stressor.

Chronic stress, also known as HPA (hypothalamic-pituitary-adrenal) stress, is a prolonged reaction to a persistent stressor, such as a demanding job or ongoing financial concerns. During chronic stress, the body releases hormones such as cortisol, which if released and not discharged can contribute to a range of health issues, including high blood pressure, heart disease, obesity, and depression.

It is important to note that not all stress is detrimental. Acute stress can actually be beneficial in certain circumstances, such as when it provides the adrenaline rush required to escape a perilous situation. Chronic stress, on the other hand, can have significant detrimental effects on health. A good way to think about stress is does this expand or contract you? I head toward challenges that may give me short-term discomfort but allow me to grow in some way. I move away from anything challenging that leaves me feeling destroyed.

Short-term stress is not necessarily bad for you.[6] In a study that tracked 30,000 adults over ten years and asked them how stressful their life was, and whether they believed that stress was harmful to their health, people who had a stressful life and firmly believed that it was bad for them had a 43 percent increase in deaths from any cause over the next decade.[7] Those with the most stressful lives who did not believe that stress was bad for them were most likely to be alive at the end of the decade. Stress isn't always the risk factor that we think it is. Stress is your body preparing for a significant metabolic outlay that may, or may not, come.

Another way to think about stress to help you avoid consequences you don't want is to imagine that you could harness the power of stress in your body to making you feel braver, more resilient, and willing to accept help from others.

In a Harvard study, before taking a test, participants were taught that the sensations they felt before it would help them prepare for the test.[8] They were told that their faster heartbeat prepared them for action, and their faster breathing was getting more oxygen to the brain. When they thought their physiological response was helpful to them, the participants felt more confident and less stressed. When people feel stressed, their blood vessels constrict, which can lead to heart disease. However, in the participants who interpreted their sensations as helpful in order to achieve their goal, their blood vessels remained relaxed.

Your physiology in states of anxiety or excitement looks like the same response. Instead of thinking your heart is racing because you are overwhelmed, might you be able to be curious about *why* your heart is racing? Could it be in service to giving you courage and confidence to carry out the task at hand?

Stress makes you hungry for support and allies. Oxytocin, the neurochemical that fine-tunes your brain's social instincts, is also known as the cuddle hormone and gets released with physical contact. It is a stress hormone motivating you to seek support, directing you to tell someone how you feel, instead of repressing your feelings. Your stress response wants you to be surrounded by people who care about you. This chemical pushes you to crave physical contact and enhances your empathy.

Stress arises when something that you care about is at stake. Stress involves physiology, feelings, emotions, thoughts, actions, and behaviors. It's the stress hormones circulating in your body and involving your need to reach out to others, or it could be anger or outrage in moments of stress. Some of these instincts are helpful and others are not. Learning about your stress instincts will help you decide what you need.

The appropriate response to *stress* is to *move*. Movement allows you to release the emotional and physical load of the stressors that happen to you. Your brain evolved to manage your complex movements. Therefore movement will shift your stress responses out of your body. The stress circuit can be broken down into:

- cause of stress
- physiological stress response
- stress residue
- appropriate action: move to recover and reset.

It is essential to differentiate between the events that *create* your stress and the lingering *effects* of the stress on you: the cause of stress and the stress residue. In the middle of those is the physiological stress response.

Let's break this down a little more. The *cause of stress* could be your demanding boss, who is never happy with your work and undermines you in front of colleagues. It could be your angry partner who works all hours and is short-tempered at home. It could be your mother always asking you when you will get married, have children, or leave your lazy slob of a partner. Or it could be even bigger toxic systems that infringe on your human rights and chip away at your ability to stay buoyant, such as racism or misogyny that you face daily. The *stress residue* is the lingering effect of the causes of stress on your brain and body. Stress is an adaptive response that has evolved to keep you safe and allow you to fight, freeze, or flee. This theory, called the general adaptation syndrome, was developed by Hans Selye,[9] a Canadian endocrinologist, and describes the idea that our nervous system reacts to stress in the same way, regardless of the stressor.

In the past, humans faced many threats to their survival, such as predators, starvation, and disease. These threats triggered the body's fight, freeze, or flight response, which is a complex physiological reaction that prepares the body to fight, freeze, or flee from danger. When the "go" part of the nervous system is activated, it causes the body to release hormones such as adrenaline and cortisol. These hormones prepare the body for action by increasing heart rate, breathing, and blood pressure; they also make the muscles tense and the senses more alert.

The fight, freeze, or flight response is a very effective way to deal with immediate threats. However, it can also be harmful if it is activated in response to nonthreatening stressors, such as an angry email or a traffic jam. Selye argued that the body responds to stress in three stages:

- **Alarm reaction**: this is the initial stage of the stress response, when the body releases hormones such as adrenaline and cortisol.
- **Resistance**: this is the second stage of the stress response, when the body tries to adapt to the stressor.
- **Exhaustion**: this is the third stage of the stress response, when the body's resources are depleted and it can no longer cope with the stressor.

If the stressor is not removed, the body can enter a state of exhaustion, which may lead to a variety of health problems, such as high blood pressure, heart disease, and anxiety.

Once upon a time the cause of stress might have been a saber-toothed tiger. As soon as you saw or heard the tiger, your brain would set off a cascade of neurological and chemical responses that activated physiological responses to give you a chance of survival. In such situations your heart beats faster and your blood pressure increases; blood is pushed into your muscles to power you for action; your muscles tense; your pain is numbed, your pupils dilate to focus on the immediate danger and blood diverts away from your digestive, reproductive, and repair systems, as there is no need for any function other than the ones that will get you out of the immediate danger. You have a strong desire for the support of others.

You don't have many options: you can run to save your life, you can try to fight the tiger or you might have to freeze and hope the tiger doesn't see you. The tiger's attention might be diverted to movement elsewhere, and you can flee when it is safe to do so.

If you successfully outrun your predator and return to your community, they will come out to protect you. You can start to release the residue of stress in your body, surrounded by the comfort of your community. You get hugged and share the story with them, and then later you collectively celebrate with a feast and you go to sleep safely, knowing that you survived another day.

You have now completed the stress circuit, used to describe the peak of the stress response to the cause of stress, and the necessary release of the residue of the chemicals in your body and brain. The release, in this instance, is running and arriving back in safety and being able to share and offload the experience with your community, with support and physical touch, comfort, and safety.

Your stress response is designed for action to get you moving out of danger and to seek the support of others. You are built for short-term stress. It keeps your brain and body sharp, motivates you toward your goals, powers you into action to seek out community and gives you the forward momentum you need to expand your experience and grow.

Once the cause of stress subsides, the "no-go" part of

your nervous system starts to reduce the stress response. Some activities will soothe your nervous system faster. These might include walking, dancing to music or being hugged and soothed by a friend. Or you could try somatic techniques, such as jiggling your whole body while tapping your fingers on your breastbone. I will guide you through this at the end of this chapter.

Under normal circumstances, once the cause of your stress is gone, the stress chemicals in your body drop, your heart rate and blood pressure normalize and your muscles release tension. Your body begins to recover.

Long-term stress, in contrast, isn't healthy. Adrenaline gives you the energy and the strength you need to speed up for a fight, freeze, or flight response. However, if your stress is continuous, this neurochemical elevates your blood pressure and narrows your blood vessels over a long period, potentially leading to heart disease and stroke.

Cortisol releases more sugar, to give you greater energy to escape or to grapple. But too much cortisol in the system creates an inflammatory response, which could cause you to become depressed or even lead to osteoporosis. How? Cortisol inhibits the production of new bone cells, which can lead to bone density loss; it also increases the activity of cells that break down bone, which can also lead to bone density loss. In addition, cortisol can weaken bones by making them more porous and less dense. It can also create fat around your belly, which promotes heart disease. Chronic stress suppresses your immune system. It gradually shortens the protective caps, or telomeres, of your chromosomes. The shortening of these structures inside your cells is thought to be strongly linked to aging.

In our modern world the causes of stress are very different from the fight, freeze, or flight scenarios described above. Rather than being short-term, they are often ongoing and cumulative. Within five minutes you can have many stress causes: receive an email with bad news about work, watch a news item about a humanitarian disaster unfolding worldwide and find out that you are already up to your overdraft limit. You sit at your laptop at home with no one to talk to, soaking up more and more micro-stresses throughout your day and taking no action with each one. What you read and take into your system makes you tighten your stomach, hold your breath, tense your neck and clench your jaw. You continue in this wound-up state throughout your day while wave after wave of micro-stresses ripple through your body and increase your levels of stress.

Now that you understand how crucial movement is to being fully human, I hope that you feel motivated to move more. And not just to move more as formal "exercise," but to move regularly throughout your day in response to micro-stresses. Movement metabolizes the intense feelings that have built up in your body and brain and need to be released. The aspiration should be for a long-term daily approach, with a range of possible movements, rather than limiting oneself to one "type" of exercise. I prefer the term "movement," as the word "exercise" conjures up the mindset of "another task I must do." Movement can include dancing in your kitchen, skipping with a rope or simply going for a walk. I enjoy a range of activities and change them up each day; they include walking the dogs, jumping on a mini-trampoline, weight training, Gyrokinesis (where the emphasis is on moving in spirals), yoga, resistance-band work, rolling around on the floor, dancing to music, roller skating, and boxing. I choose what I do according to my feelings and energy for the day. If I don't have much energy, I will break up my working day with some mobility movement on the floor or I will go for a walk to allow my eyes to soften from their fixed state and to rest my brain.

As you move more and sense the change in your emotional and physical state, you will start to form positive habits that will make you look forward to moving every day. But most importantly, you will start to feel good!

Shaking lesson

Shaking is a natural response to your body to release itself from a fixed state, which could be bad news, a shock or a fright, or if you have been stuck in one position for a long time. If you have a dog, you will have seen it shake when it experiences extreme excitement or fear—shaking releases a surge of chemicals in the body to prepare dogs for action. The shaking allows them to transition from the excited state into a more settled one. You can do the same thing.

You have already practiced a lying-down version in the restorative rocking lesson (see page 39) in Chapter 1. This is my standing version:

1   Stand and place your feet sit-bone distance apart.
2   Let your arms dangle by your sides. Let your knees bend slightly, and press your feet into the floor.
3   Now start to slide your shoulder blades up to your ears and back down, and pick up the pace slowly as if you are shrugging your shoulders up and down.

4 Let this movement travel through your pelvis and
   legs. The movement should start to feel like you are
   bouncing slowly on a trampoline, without your feet
   leaving the floor.
5 Find an effortless pace, and let the movement go
   through you, like wobbly jelly. The movement should
   feel easy and pleasant.
6 Once you have that going, you can slowly rotate your
   chest, upper body, and arms from one side to the
   other. Your head will come along for the ride. The
   twist is from the belly upward, so the pelvis will
   move. Please don't keep it rigid. The movement is
   more from the upper body turning as you jiggle.
7 I usually play a nice piece of music—R&B works for
   me—and jiggle for the whole song. Once you gently
   stop, notice how you feel: tingly in the fingers, arms
   hanging effortlessly? Has your noisy mind quieted
   down?

What you have learned in this chapter

- As humans, we are designed to move. The best
  exercise for your brain is movement. There is a
  direct link between the body and mind in the brain's
  structure. Movement, thinking, and planning,
  and control of involuntary bodily functions are
  interconnected.
- Your nervous system, including your brain, evolved
  to move you in your environment to sense and
  interact with it.
- Movement improves your mood, combats anxiety

and depression, and reduces your risk of age-related brain diseases.

- Movement can undo the damage caused by stress— release the residue of stress with micro-movements to enable the chemicals to move out of your body and brain.
- Think about more movement in and throughout your day: stand sometimes instead of sitting, bike to the store, walk up and down the stairs, encourage walk-and-talk meetings.
- If you want to change your emotional state, *move!*

Now put the book down and go outside to do nothing other than gently let this information sink in. In the next chapter we look at rest, and why this is critical to being fully human.

6

Rest

Each person deserves a day away in which no problems are confronted, no solutions searched for. Each of us needs to withdraw from the cares which will not withdraw from us.

Maya Angelou, *Letter to My Daughter*[1]

When I first started practicing yoga I would always leave the class before that bit at the end where you do nothing but lie there. It's called Savasana or corpse pose. It felt like dead time to me, when I could spend the time on *getting things done* instead.

I have always striven to work hard: I am the daughter of immigrants to this country and grew up in a South Asian household. My parents worked hard and instilled the same work ethic in me. They had no safety net of an extended family in the same country and had to keep working, no matter what else was going on. My first job was working as a hairdresser, aged fourteen, and I have earned my own money ever since. I have never stopped working.

Work is now so central to our idea of who we are that many people find it disorientating when they no longer have a job. When the pandemic came along and we had to collectively stop doing things in the way we used to, it was the first time we had faced who we are and what we do, without the concept of going out to work defining us. Among my clients, the older male ones found it extremely hard to be at home, in what they felt was their wives' domain. Professional women who had been busy for decades no longer had to commute, and once the home-schooling pressures had calmed down, they could magic up time to practice yoga or enjoy spending little pockets of time with their children that wasn't fully scheduled. Although many women complained about being the snack provider, I also know many couples who reconfigured their family life, once it became apparent that the mother had been doing all the heavy lifting at home.

For many people, the pandemic opened their eyes to how relentlessly exhausting their lives had been. Of course there was a lot of fear and anxiety, because none of us knew how things would pan out for us, for our loved ones and for society at large. But it was a chance to imagine a different type of life as we eventually moved on from it. When you are busy with commuting, working, and life admin, you often don't have the mental space to consider who you really want to be at different stages of your life.

Often our idea of ourselves is formed as a child at school, and then we are off at breakneck speed growing into that idea. As I grew up in my South Asian household, the cliché wish of Asian parents wanting their children to become doctors and lawyers was very real. Both are considered consistent professions where you will always be employed, and they have a status attached to them. I have a few clients who did what their parents wanted them to do: married the person they were encouraged to marry, had the required number of children and a promising career. Then, when they reach midlife, they realized they had lived their lives for others. Most of us have no pauses to reflect and consider, "Is this who I still want to be?" Without time for self-reflection, how do you gauge where you are and where you want to go? How do you shift your way through your changing values and dreams? Rest is equally as important as action.

Rest is such an alien concept in the culture that we live in. We often push ourselves until we break. I watch my friends who are mothers drive themselves relentlessly throughout their lives, keeping up with impossible schedules and, with the best intentions, pushing their children in the same way. They become an endless stream of nurturing and entertainment and serve as an emotional container for their family. But all this extra work leaves them feeling despondent, besides already being exhausted with their careers. How is it possible to deliver on all fronts constantly throughout our lives? It is impossible—something has to give, and that is usually your physical and mental health.

Case study: Nicola

Nicola was referred to me by her therapist. She had reached a point where she felt physically and emotionally stuck. She had experienced fertility issues, financial worries and complex family dynamics, which caused her ongoing emotional pain. Like many women who manage a career and a home life, she was exhausted and had hit a wall that her regular good habits of eating nutritious food, regular exercise and eight hours of sleep were not helping her to break through.

She noticed that as well as feeling exhausted, she was unhappy, overwhelmed and despondent about her life. She told me that she felt disconnected from herself. She hurtled through her day, reacting to events as they came up. There was no time to think, to pause and to consider. She had no rest.

Nicola had a hopeful face, and I could see that she was doing her very best, but her forging-ahead strategies were no longer working. I could see that she was holding herself unconfidently. Her rounded shoulders pulled her into herself. This influenced her breathing, which was short and shallow.

We started with small movements that engaged her interest in her current state. How did she feel when she lay on the floor? It was often a relief that she didn't have to do one more thing. Where in her body could she feel her exhaustion? It was in her sunken chest. Where did she feel her rising panic about the future? It was in her belly, which churned with anxiety.

Slowly, over twelve weeks, we unpicked the tension in her body so that she could fully accommodate her breath. She felt elated when she worked out the puzzle of the movement guidance that I gave her: how do you get one foot to trace around the shape of your other foot? The more you bend, sway and soften, the easier it becomes. Working things out in a considered way gave Nicola the confidence to try new things. She learned to rest, to deal with her feelings as they arose and to calm her system before she began constructive conversations with her partner. She felt a reconnection with the things in life that brought her joy. She felt confident enough to take control of her relationship and make choices that were right for her, rather than trying to keep the peace at home. She felt more robust and able to think clearly.

Nicola now stands tall, finding a dynamic posture at any given time. She is doing things she had only dreamed of, including enrolling in a creative-writing course. She has plans that expand her idea of herself outside her family and work. This gives her agency as a person, which acknowledges her personal needs. Introducing frequent counter-practices to her micro-stresses throughout the day has allowed her system to rest, recalibrate, and restore. This has enabled her to see how she wasn't using her energy to improve her life, but had lain at modern motherhood's sacrificial altar. You cannot make sound decisions from an exhausted brain. Breaking yourself to serve others is not a sustainable strategy.

Resting and noticing

Women take on many roles: colleague, partner, mother, daughter, sister. And in our busy lives, where we have many things to manage, we constantly fail when we can't do everything. The trope of having it all was a misrepresentation of the feminist movement of the 1970s, arguing that equality between the genders would come only if the preconditions for emancipation included childcare, legal abortion, and equal pay. Feminism was co-opted by self-help and lifestyle magazines and mutated from a collective approach to an individual policy. Women were guided on how to have it all, with recommendations on what to buy and what to wear to help get them there. The myth of the blow-dried, sharp-suited, high-heeled superwoman with a briefcase in one hand and a baby on her hip was born.

Doing everything to the same standard always is just not possible. In an ideal scenario, you would have the time to move smoothly from one type of role or activity to another. In between, you would rest from the focus of the current activity and prepare for the following next activity. The transitions between activities are as important as the activity itself. Marking these transitions with rituals is an important part of signifying the end of one thing and the beginning of another.

Noticing and tending to how you feel throughout your day is a critical reflection to enable you to process your feelings, emotions, thoughts, actions, and behaviors. For example, you are working on a crucial pitch document at your desk. An email alert arrives and you check your inbox to find an email reminding you that you need to pay a big, overdue tax bill. Even with the strongest will in the world, most people would find it challenging to stay in the creative zone.

Sitting at your desk trying to switch your thoughts back to the task and typing through it probably won't help you to focus. A good strategy would be to leave your desk, get some fresh air and form a strategy for addressing your tax payments. Once you have a plan of action, which could be to call the tax office first thing in the morning, you follow on with a walk around the park and let your eyes soft-focus on the grass, or the leaves of the trees, so that they become less tense. Allow your breathing to slow down to a more even pace. Now you have recovered and reset. When you return to your desk, switch off your email and start writing again, safely back in your creative zone.

Tending to yourself in real time, particularly in the digital age where work has no end, is critical to prevent the buildup of your responses to stressful events throughout the day that accumulate and create inflammation in your body. Managing yourself to deal with your micro-stresses in real time will prevent you from burning out, feeling perpetually stressed and anxious, overwhelmed, despondent, or angry at the impossible expectations heaped upon you.

Here is how I ensure that I deal with the things that come up during the day when I'm teaching others: I tend to wake up around 7 a.m. and I prefer more strenuous movement in the mornings; this could be walking, jumping on my mini-trampoline, exercising with weights, or doing anything vigorous and strengthening. I have a busy clinic with clients throughout my day. When I started working online, I gave myself five minutes between each client. My rationale was that now I was entirely online, I no longer had to make time for the commute from one client to another. The five-minute gap between clients would give me enough time to switch off from one meeting and start the next.

However, I often felt exhausted and emotionally wrenched by my clients' problems. What I wasn't doing was dealing with the emotional load that builds up on me from observing the suffering of others. I am human, after all. Other people's stories influence how I feel, and I learned to metabolize them through me. Metabolism, in this sense, means converting my feelings into action so that they move through me.

To process the intensity of teaching on a one-to-one basis, I now have built-in release rituals between each client. I either jump on my trampoline to music, breathe fully into my lungs, lie on the floor or roll out any tension in my body. The limit to how many clients I can see, one after the other, is two clients in the morning and, when that is done, I leave my studio and engage in something that gives me a mental break. I use that time to cook, garden, clean, sew, play with my dogs, chat with my partner who works from home or pop out for a walk on the beach, and I make a point of having spontaneous conversations with others.

Ideally, my release rituals include movement, breath, daylight, nature, creativity, and social connection. I favor any ritual that allows my mind to wander without focus. In the midafternoon I often practice a guided somatic meditation called NSDR (Non-Sleep Deep Rest),[2] focusing on noticing my sensations.

All of this makes me better at letting go and not over-thinking my work, which takes up much of my brain, including prepping for classes or clients, and holding the space within a class or session and the actual teaching. I realized that if I didn't let my brain release from its intense focus, I often felt weighted down by other people's prob-lems. It left me exhausted at the end of the day, and my mind would be thinking and planning even when I switched off my light to go to sleep.

It took me a long time to get here. At many times in my life, self-reflection has felt like an uncomfortable engage-ment and, looking back, I realize that moving fast during my downtime was an attempt to outrun my feelings. It can be helpful to experience the discomfort of reflection: not to dwell on, or beat ourselves up over, decisions we have made, but to learn and grow from them. The key learning is that I did not allow myself pauses to do that, because I did not value the importance of rest.

Why do we revere the idea of busyness to the detriment of our own physical and mental health?

Busyness

The word "lazy" is thought to derive from the low-middle German *lasich*, which means "weak," or from the Old English *lesu*, which means "evil" or "false"—being lazy means that you lack discipline or are weak or morally corrupt. This idea remains strong in our culture: lazy people are deemed feckless and failures.

The concept that work is good for the soul came from the Puritans, an arm of Christianity that believed God chose hard workers for redemption and that being industrious was a sign of piety. Conversely, if someone couldn't motivate themselves or failed to meet their responsibilities, they were unworthy of salvation. This idea leaves little sympathy for those who struggled or failed in any way.

The Puritans migrated their ideas to the United States. This idea of hard work twinned with self-worth underpinned the newly emerging societies to give them a sense of purpose. The concept of hardworking people being morally superior became politically useful, and was used to motivate settlers in harsh lands and, subsequently, enslaved people. A new religious idea was formed around the idea that work improved character, that suffering was ethically righteous and that enslaved people would be rewarded in heaven for their diligence. Working without complaint was seen as virtuous. Conversely, lazy enslaved people were deemed morally corrupt. Valuing hard work above all else was also integral to fueling the capitalist dream throughout the twentieth century. And the idea that idle time for workers will lead to riots and social unrest still permeates the political and economic systems that govern us.

The cult of busyness teaches us that being busy is superior to resting. It tells us that if we're not constantly doing something, then we're lazy or unproductive. This mindset can lead us to mistrust our own feelings. When we're tired, we reach for a coffee instead of listening to our bodies' need for rest. When we're feeling sad, we go shopping instead of allowing ourselves to experience our emotions. We start to believe there's always a product we can buy to fix our problems, even when the "problem" is simply being human. We outsource our soothing with external solutions, when the answer lies within.

The human brain is simply incapable of focusing continuously for eight hours a day, so how did we end up with this expectation? The eight-hour working day is a hangover from the industrial age, when manual workers slogged for between ten and sixteen hours a day—and often six days a week—because factories ran for twenty-four hours. In the late eighteenth century the "eight-hour-day movement" looked to improve the working week. However, it wasn't until 1914 that Ford Motors reduced the working day to eight hours and increased pay, which saw productivity double. The new working day significantly improved upon previous conditions in the manufacturing age, but it's not working well for us now in our brain-fueled knowledge economy.

A study showed that the average US worker is productive for two hours and fifty-three minutes a day; the rest of the time is spent chatting, in meetings and browsing online. However, driven by various pressures, a substantial number of US workers feel obligated to be physically present at work even when unwell. A striking 77 percent of respondents admitted to working while sick, with diverse reasons underlying this behavior. Heavy workloads emerged as the primary culprit for a third of these employees, followed by concerns about job security and the need to save vacation days for childcare.[3,4] There are many reasons why people might engage in presenteeism. Some people may feel pressure to come to work even when they are sick, for fear of losing their job or not being seen as a team player. Others may feel they cannot afford to take time off work, even if they are not feeling well. Presenteeism is linked to stress, anxiety, and depression.

A tendency to focus on always being productive views the human being as a machine, its sole purpose to work continuously, stopping only to refuel and sleep. I worked in an office for one period of my life. Before this, I had mainly worked for myself. I struggled to understand why I couldn't wander off when I had done enough. The pretense of appearing to be busy for a full working day, five days a week, was the element that I found most challenging about the job. How to appear to be earning my salary, hour after hour, was quite a mental burden. I left that job, hoping never to return to a formal work setting again. It was not conducive to my mental health.

At the forefront of innovative working models once again, Ford announced in 2021 that its employees could permanently work from home after the pandemic, while other companies were ordering their employees back to the office. Ford's office buildings have become collaborative spaces for meetings and projects, but its employees work from home for focused work. In a recent study of trialing a four-day week without losing wages, most companies reported that productivity and performance stayed the same. In addition, employees said they felt less burnout, and the additional time enabled them to manage their lives better.[5]

We are stuck in this outmoded idea of presenteeism: being at your desk for the allocated time of your contract ensures that you are paid your fee. And yet there are so many distractions in the workplace that interrupt your ability to pay attention, including navigating other people, meetings, noise and open-plan offices that offer no quiet time and add to the mental fatigue. What if chatting with colleagues, reading, or thinking about things other than work allows your brain to recalibrate? What if resting from your focus through your day improves the quality of your thinking?

We all know that a little bit of stress can improve our focus, but too much sustained stress—such as impossible deadlines, a never-ending to-do list, a demanding boss or a toxic workplace—impairs our ability to focus. This is because the front part of our brain, the prefrontal cortex, decides what to pay cognitive attention to, coordinating inputs from other brain areas and diverting our visual attention to what we focus on. When we multitask, our brain splits its attention between one task and then another, rather than focusing on everything. There may be a few people who can successfully multitask, but for most of us it is physiologically impossible.

When mental fatigue sets in, you might feel sleepy and unmotivated and your performance deteriorates. Your attitude and your mood are affected. If you notice that you are easily distracted from focusing on the task at hand, it might mean that it is time for a break, to allow your brain to release itself from a state of deep focus.

Intermittent resting

You've probably heard of the circadian rhythm: twenty-four-hour cycles that form the internal body's clock; they coordinate the cascade of processes that occur at different times throughout the day and night. The circadian rhythm influences every aspect of biological function, including body temperature, mood and alertness.

You might not have heard of ultradian rhythms, also known as the basic rest-and-activity cycle; these are biological patterns in the internal body which are shorter than the circadian rhythm of twenty-four hours, and which cycle throughout the day. Just as in sleep, where you enter ninety-minute cycles of REM (rapid eye movement) and NREM (non-rapid eye movement) sleep, so your body runs a similar process throughout the day. Your body and brain burn through oxygen, glucose, and other energetic fuels during their focused work. Your heart rate, hormonal levels, muscle tension, and alertness all peak at the first part of the cycle. Metabolic waste, which is the by-product of your mental and physical activity, builds up and you begin to experience this as stress.

At around 90–120 minutes you start to get easily distracted, you may have trouble keeping attention, the signals from your body start dialing up and you begin to feel fidgety, irritable, hungry, or tired. Your productivity starts to wane as you experience declining energy. Your body needs some downtime. It must regenerate and rebalance, flush out debris and toxins, and repair damaged tissue. Your brain requires a break from taking in information and needs to process, create essential connections and arrive at solutions. It's a rest-and-activity cycle to allow your system to recalibrate. If you can attune yourself to these rhythms, you can ride on the wave of your body's intelligent alertness and sleepiness cycles and plan your work accordingly.

I have been working like this for a while and have found it a compassionate way to organize my day. I limit the time spent on one work segment to ninety minutes, and when that time is up, I do something else. The more I work like this, the easier it gets to focus on one thing. Give yourself twenty minutes of downloading time between your focus time, which enables the brain to process the information you have been digesting; the rest allows you to consolidate and transition smoothly onto the next activity.

Whereas previously I skipped from project to project and felt wrung out at the end of the day, I now plan my focused work first thing in the morning. I take a break for twenty minutes or so, then I plan my next round of ninety minutes, and that's it for my focused type of work. I might have another burst in the afternoon. Generally I aim for two sets of ninety-minute focused work. Ideally, my twenty-minute break is an entirely different type of activity and is not desk- or device-bound. The less focused work is usually life admin or planning lessons, where I am trying movement out on the mat. I might also practice breathwork or meditate, and build in an afternoon nap of twenty minutes as often as possible. Ensure that you choose a different type of work from sitting at a laptop and paying focused attention. I do realize that my working day is completely different from most other people's.

How to find the start of your ninety minutes? Keep a journal to see when you feel most alert in the morning. My morning cycles hit me at 9 a.m. and 11:30 a.m. I don't waste time doing the jobs I don't like then, such as paying bills; I do the things I want to do and that are creative—the work that gives me meaning—such as teaching, practicing, researching, and writing.

How to fit this into your day in an office? Let's assume you start at 9 a.m. Notice how alert you feel at 9:30 a.m. and, if this is your time, ring-fence the next ninety minutes to work. Take a break at 11 a.m., leave your desk, walk around the office, climb some stairs, talk to your colleagues or get a coffee. At 11:20 a.m. you are back at your desk, and this is a good time to tend to emails, office admin, and all the other things that never seem to end. Leave your desk and walk at lunchtime, and eat away from your desk if possible. After lunch, sit with some paper away from your desk and plan what you will do with the rest of the afternoon. Leave yourself enough time at the end of the day to review, gather your thoughts and plan for the following day. If you can, close your eyes and focus on breathing as you allow your feet to ground themselves into the floor. I will cover more of this in the next part of the book.

This ideal scenario makes no room for meetings, traveling and all the other unplanned events that land in your lap. But it gives you an idea of how you can apply focus and recover from the focus in cycles throughout your day. My advice is to move toward this way of working by changing one thing at a time. Even if you manage one round of uninterrupted focused work and remember to leave your seat several times a day more than you do now, you are moving in the direction of tending to your nervous system.

Rest counters action, and prepares you for your next bout of action. You cannot run your nervous system continuously and still be effective: rest and action work together to give you a balanced system.

To illustrate the importance of rest for peak performance, we can look at a study of violin students at the Berlin Conservatory in 1993.[6] The researchers were interested in identifying the factors that contributed to outstanding performance in these students. One of the most striking findings of the study was that the best students were also the ones who took the most breaks. They didn't practice for hours on end without stopping. Instead they took regular breaks to rest and recharge. This allowed them to stay focused and motivated and to avoid burnout.

The study's findings suggest that rest is essential for peak performance. When we're well rested, we're able to focus better, learn more effectively and make better decisions. We're also less likely to experience stress, anxiety, and burnout. The takeaway from this is that if you're looking to improve your performance, be sure to get enough rest. Take breaks throughout the day and make sure you're getting restful sleep. Your body and mind will thank you for it.

The more successful students practiced more deliberately, with total concentration, paying attention to what they were doing and observing where they could improve. They sensed that these sessions reinforced their idea of the great musicians they would become. The researchers also found that deliberate practice is effortful and can only be sustained for a few hours daily. The time spent on deliberate practice is an amount they can recover from. Their sessions involved periods of ninety minutes with a thirty-minute break in between. Too much practice and they sustained injuries.

Additionally, they found that the top performers slept for an hour more than other students. They slept in the afternoon, after which they practiced for one more block of ninety minutes. This worked out to about four hours of focused attention a day. The rest of the time wasn't spent being idle; they did their homework and other practice, but the focused work was limited to these shorter practices. They applied themselves according to the available mental and physical resources for daily effortful practice.

A study conducted in the 1950s surveyed scientists' hours worked versus the number of articles they produced.[7] Scientists who worked ten to twenty hours per week had a good ratio versus pieces produced. Those who worked twenty-five hours a week were no more productive than those who spent five hours a week working. Those who worked thirty-five hours a week were half as productive as their colleagues' twenty hours a week. The scientists who spent sixty-plus hours a week were the least effective. The most successful scientists were working between four and six hours a day.

Scientists, scholars, and writers follow this short and focused working pattern. For example, the naturalist Charles Darwin and the writer Charles Dickens recorded that they worked four hours per day, interrupted by walking when they had to think. Darwin even had a thinking path that he walked along when he had to resolve complex problems.

We focus far too much on the *doing* and not so much on the *resting* from doing. I see this again and again in my clients. A typical pattern is that they get up and work out, get their children ready and out of the house. They then push on through the day without stopping again until bedtime: tapping furiously on a keyboard with no breaks, lunch eaten at their desk, online food shopping organized on the phone between meetings, meals eaten watching Netflix. There is no time to rest and reflect. So it is unsurprising that they cannot sleep, have digestive issues and suffer from anxiety, stress, and burnout.

Many studies show that resting consolidates learning. Your mind at rest replays memories, plans for the future and imagines different scenarios. Fifteen minutes of resting during the day, with your eyes closed, can significantly boost your memory, with the effects lasting for up to one week.

The difference between rest and sleep

Regular rest is needed throughout the day to allow you to recover from mental and physical activity, and sleep is your twenty-four-hour reset for the good health of your brain and body. Let's look at how our sleep cycles between REM (rapid eye movement) and NREM (non-rapid eye movement).

NREM sleep further subdivides into four stages, increasing the depth of your sleep. In the first two stages you shift from wakefulness into light sleep, your heart rate decreases and your body temperature and electrical brain waves slow down. Stages three and four are where your brain erupts with powerful brain waves and your immune and cardiovascular systems are recharged. These later stages of sleep are where the consolidation of memories happens and becomes fixed in the brain's architecture.

REM sleep is where the brain wave activity speeds up and you have vivid dreams. This is where emotional regulation, creativity, the processing of information and problem-solving occur.

This interplay between REM and NREM sleep happens in the standard ninety-minute cycle, but the ratio of REM to NREM sleep changes as you move through the night. For example, in the first half of the night you have deeper NREM sleep, but as you go through the second half of the night you have more REM sleep and lighter NREM sleep.

Missing out on any part of this cycling means that you don't enjoy the full benefits that sleep can give you—and it does this every twenty-four hours. The benefits include restoration, brain processing, and memory allocation, and novel solutions to complex problems: neural connections

are linked and strengthened, and the ones that are not reinforced will fall away.

During the 1940s the average person in the US enjoyed
seven to nine hours of sleep per day on average; in 2023, it was
six hours and forty-eight minutes.[8] So why aren't we getting
enough sleep? Demanding jobs, rolling news, social media,
film-streaming, and other aspects of our lifestyle are all cited
as sleep stealers.

What happens when you are sleep-deprived? As well as
suffering from poor memory and poor judgment, there
are even more serious repercussions. Short sleep duration is
linked to a higher risk of cancer, with shift workers showing
higher rates than those who work regular office hours. If
you sleep for five hours or less every night, you have a 50
percent likelihood of being obese, because of the rise of
the hunger hormone in the system. Tired people suffer from
sustained stress linked to higher infection rates. You are at
increased risk of developing type 2 diabetes and cardiovascular disease. You are more likely to suffer from depression,
anxiety, emotional distress, and mood disorders. In cases of
severe mental illness, there is almost always sleep disruption.

Stabilizing sleep can alleviate the symptoms. Our relationship to sleep needs to be regeared: instead of considering
sleep as something that has to be fixed, we need to prioritize sleep as a necessary part of our life, rather than one
that is squished in when we are at the end of our tether. For
example, many of us take daily stimulants to stay awake and
drink alcohol to numb our sleep. However, once you start to
include rest throughout your day, your sleep will improve.

Rest lesson

Try the following for a twenty-minute break:

1 Lie on the floor with your legs extended and your
   arms by your side. Let there be space between your
   arms and your torso.
2 Notice the weight of your bones on the floor.
3 Start to notice your breath and how your whole self
   accommodates it; what parts of you move in time to
   your breathing?
4 Notice which of your ribs connect with the floor.
   The next time you inhale, allow the ribs that contact
   the ground to press into the floor gradually and, as
   you exhale, let the ribs slowly release their pressure
   from the floor.
5 Repeat this a few times, but keep making it softer
   and softer so that it feels as if your breathing and the
   increase and decrease of the pressure of your ribs on
   the floor are the same action. The breath smoothly
   transitions into the movement.
6 As soon as you notice that you are not fully engaged
   or are tired, take a rest from the deep concentration
   and try it again after you have rested.
7 You can now move on to your shoulder blades, the
   back of your skull, pelvis, calves, and heels. Again,
   take your time, and rest after focusing on one part
   before you move on to the next.
8 Rest from all this and notice how your contact with
   the floor has changed in resting. Has it? The sensation
   might be subtle, but regular somatic practice will
   start to fine-tune your range of sensations.

What you have learned in this chapter

- Mother Nature has given you the easiest way to recharge and reboot your system every twenty-four hours, with sleep.
- Allowing your mind to rest without stimulus enables it to replay memories, future-plan, and imagine different scenarios. Doing so consolidates learning and increases creativity.
- You have ninety-minute/twenty-minute rhythms of activity and rest throughout the day. If you plan around the peaks and troughs of brain performance, you will get your focused work done more effectively.
- Sleep has different cycles throughout the night and it is important to allow time to complete them all to enjoy the full benefits—including emotional regulation.
- Give sleep and rest equal billing to action and productivity, so that you can balance your system and function at your optimum.

We have covered much information on the importance of rest and the crucial role of sleep. You probably feel a little tired. Put the book down and enjoy a twenty-minute break from thinking. Go for a walk, curl up on the sofa or chat with someone in the real world. In the next chapter we will cover how your food nourishes your brain, the gut–brain connection and the importance of being in nature.

7

Nourishment

Eat food. Not too much. Mainly plants.
Michael Pollan, *In Defense of Food: An Eater's Manifesto*[1]

I worked in a health-food shop when I was nineteen. It was one of the best educations I have had. I learned about how food can be medicine, and I learned how to eat unprocessed foods as close to their natural state as possible. I stopped eating meat because of the antibiotics used in meat production at the time, and I felt squeamish about food production. I learned how to use herbs to soothe. I learned that echinacea, a flowering plant, is commonly used to treat colds and flu; it is thought to boost the immune system and help the body fight off infection. I learned that garlic has been used for centuries for its medicinal properties; it is thought to have antibiotic, antifungal, and antiviral properties. I deliberately include garlic when I cook, especially in the colder months.

The knowledge that you can use food as medicine has stayed with me all my life. My mother used to cook from scratch, as it was cheaper to do so and you knew what ingredients you were putting into your pot. Occasionally she would let us have a fast-food burger. We thought it was a treat and a break from

eating homemade food. Children are so ungrateful sometimes, aren't they? Now fast food is more than an occasional
"treat." Consumers buying takeout food and home deliveries
increased by 30 percent, year on year, in 2021. In the US, the
market has more than doubled during the Covid-19 pandemic.
The fast-food and takeout industry in the US is currently
valued at approximately $320 billion to $387.5 billion, making
it a significant segment of the US economy.[2]

There is so much information on what to eat, how to
eat and when to eat; yet still we are confused about how to
nourish our bodies. We zone in on the latest fads reported
in the press because, in a world with so many choices, we
are desperate to find the answer to what to eat in order
to be healthy. We have specific diets: vegetarian, vegan,
pescatarian, paleo, low-GI, sugar-free, gluten-free, and
dairy-free. It seems that the more information we can tap
into, the more confused we become.

A large study that linked various other studies across
sixty years found that plant-based food protects against most
chronic diseases, compared to animal-based foods.[3] Whole-
grain-based foods are slightly more protective; highly refined
grains are not good for us. Dairy foods came out as neutral.
Red and processed meat increased our risk. This information is probably consistent with what you already know. But
the diet industry makes it so much more complex than that.
Even I sometimes get confused about what I should include
in my diet. However, I continue to try to eat plant-based
foods and now, with all the new information about the gut
microbiome (see page 171), I try to include a diverse range
of plant-based foods in my diet.

Your brain and nervous system are complex organs that

require a variety of nutrients to function properly. Eating a nutritious diet is essential for maintaining brain health and cognitive function. Some of the most important nutrients for the brain and nervous system include:

- omega-3 fatty acids, which are essential for the development and function of the brain and nervous system.[4] They help to protect the brain from damage and improve cognitive function. Good sources of omega-3 fatty acids include fatty fish, such as salmon, tuna, and mackerel, walnuts, and flaxseeds.
- folate, which is a B vitamin that is essential to produce new nerve cells.[5] It is also important for the formation of myelin, the protective sheath that surrounds nerve cells. Good sources of folate include leafy green vegetables, such as spinach and broccoli, citrus fruit, and legumes.
- vitamin B12, which is another B vitamin that is essential for the nervous system.[6] It helps to produce energy and maintain the health of nerve cells. Good sources of vitamin B12 include meat, poultry, fish, eggs, and dairy products.
- iron, which helps to transport oxygen to the brain.[7] Low iron levels can lead to fatigue, difficulty concentrating, and other cognitive problems. Good sources of iron include red meat, poultry, fish, beans, and lentils.
- zinc, which is essential to help protect the brain from damage and improve cognitive function. Good sources of zinc include red meat, poultry, seafood, beans, and nuts.

In addition to these, the brain and nervous system also need a variety of other nutrients, such as vitamins A, C, and E, magnesium and potassium. These can be found in a variety of fruit, in fish such as salmon, tuna, and mackerel, and in walnuts and flaxseeds.

According to Tim Spector, a British epidemiologist and professor of genetic epidemiology at King's College London, you should eat at least thirty different plants per week. This is based on his research, which has shown that people who eat a variety of plants have a healthier gut microbiome (see page 171) and a lower risk of chronic diseases, such as heart disease, stroke, and cancer.[8]

I eat a diverse range of plants as part of my diet, but *thirty* different plants was quite the challenge, until I found out that the definition of a plant is anything that comes from one—including fruit, vegetables, legumes, nuts, seeds, spices, herbs, and whole grains. Spector recommends that you eat a variety of plants from all different colors of the rainbow, as each color contains different nutrients. For example, red fruit and vegetables are good sources of antioxidants, while green leafy vegetables are beneficial sources of vitamins A and C.

If you're not sure how to get thirty different plants into your diet, here are a few tips:

- Explore seasonal fruit and vegetables every week. This is a good way to experiment with tastes and try new recipes.
- Add nuts and seeds to your snacks. Nuts and seeds are a great source of nutrients and can help you feel full.
- Cook with whole grains, which are a good source of fiber and nutrients.

- Fermented foods are also a great source of probiotics, which are beneficial for your gut health.

In addition to eating foods that nourish the nervous system, I am also interested in how our modern lives impact upon it. In particular the emergence of chemically complex foods, called ultra-processed foods (UPFs), and how they can disrupt the nervous system.

The trouble with UPFs

First, let's look at how the food industry has changed the way many people now eat. A typical day starts with a sugary cereal or something pastry-based for breakfast, followed by a sandwich at lunchtime, a sweet snack in the afternoon, and a frozen dinner with wine in the evening. Because of the demands on our time, we have moved away from cooking fresh food at home. The problem with this is the added ingredients found in commercially processed food to make them fresh for longer, and to encourage you to buy them.

UPFs contain ingredients that you wouldn't find in your kitchen; they undergo extensive processing and contain many additives, preservatives, and artificial ingredients, in combinations that you wouldn't usually put together. They are often high in refined sugars, unhealthy fats, and additives such as flavor enhancers and artificial colors. Commonly consumed UPFs are sugary drinks, packaged snacks, fast foods, frozen meals, and breakfast cereals. If you turn over your store-bought packaged food and look at the ever-growing list of ingredients, I can guarantee you probably wouldn't recognize what most of them are.

How you feel can influence the foods that you eat, and what you eat can influence how you feel. Adults who regularly eat junk food are at an increased risk of developing depression and dementia. The chance of developing these conditions is impacted by the quality of the food consumed over a lifespan.

A study called SMILES (Supporting the Modification of lifestyle in Lowered Emotional States) looked at diet and mood.[9] It took place over a few years, with 176 people who suffered from moderate to severe depression. They entered one part of these into a dietary support group, and one-third of those people recovered from their major depression. Of the group who were offered just social support, only eight people recovered.

Our modern diet is leading to increased obesity and mental-health issues. Your brain is geared toward pleasurable activities. When you engage in anything that gives you pleasure—from socializing or having sex to eating delicious food—your brain's reward system releases dopamine, a neurotransmitter with strong responses to rewards and positive motivation. When you eat junk foods like UPFs, with their high-fat, sugary or salty tastes, these flavors are often combined to make the food even more compelling. If you consistently eat junk foods, your brain adapts by producing more receptors for dopamine. As more dopamine receptors are stimulated, you must eat more of these foods to experience the same pleasurable feelings. This means that your brain urges you to eat more of these foods, causing you to crave them.

When you overindulge in these foods, you start to impair the part of the brain that governs decision-making, your prefrontal cortex. UPFs are particularly concerning, because they are engineered to have the optimal combination of fat, sugars, and salts, which creates a pleasurable sensory experience. This combination can stimulate reward centers in your brain, leading to cravings and a desire for more. This hyper-palatable quality of UPFs can override normal hunger and satiety, making it difficult to stop eating when you feel full.

I have an insatiable desire for certain foods—I have a serious issue with chips. I find the salt and fat content of them so compelling that I will eat a big packet without thinking. I cannot have them in the house, and I only buy them when others are around. Having people around me who might disapprove of my chip addiction moderates my behavior. My genes were tested many years ago, and a nutritionist interpreted the results for me: it turns out that not only do I have an addiction and overeating gene, but I also respond well to exercise. This means that I have a propensity to these things, but I have managed my natural inclinations through lifestyle choices. I have naturally been drawn to exercise daily to manage my emotions, which means that I somehow knew what my body wanted and that I needed to self-regulate with movement. The body is inherent wisdom in action—all you need to do is listen.

UPFs are heavily advertised, and food advertising often twins the food with an emotional state. A common theme is to eat foods that make you feel good and use them as external soothing mechanisms. You might have heard the phrase "wine-o'clock," referring to a time of day when work is over and you can kick back by pouring yourself a glass of wine to de-stress. But regular alcohol consumption, for some people, can increase stress levels by releasing cortisol even when they are not drinking. A globally well-known burger commercial links spending time with your divorced dad on alternate weekends with a trip to the burger place. The implication is that the perfect combination of store-bought fats, sugars, and salts will soothe your feelings of confusion over familial loyalties. The commercial plays on the idea that unhealthy food can be a form of comfort, an idea promoted by the fast-food industry.

Constant exposure to food advertisements and the convenience of these foods can contribute to their addictive nature. The message is that the foods you buy to make yourself feel better, or to show love to others, will dampen your stress and loneliness, your sense of feeling unworthy or unloved. But eating to soothe yourself externalizes the internal response to your feelings. It is fleeting and disrupts the proper functioning of your nervous system.

How do ultra-processed foods affect your nervous system? UPFs can disrupt the balance of neurotransmitters in the brain, such as dopamine (which motivates you toward rewards) and serotonin (feelings of contentment). When you experience disruption to these systems, it can lead to mood swings, cravings, and mental-health issues such as anxiety and depression. Consumption of UPFs has also been linked to chronic inflammation in your body, including in your brain, impairing the functioning of and communication between your neurons, which can affect memory, cognitive function, and mood regulation.

UPFs can also disrupt the balance of beneficial bacteria in the gut. Your gut–brain axis is the two-way communication between your gastrointestinal tract and your nervous system, including your brain. Any imbalance can influence neurotransmitter production, immune system function and, as already noted, your mental health.

What is your gut microbiome?

The gut microbiome is a collection of microorganisms in the gastrointestinal tract—a passageway about nine meters long that runs from your mouth to your anus. It is a part of your digestive system that includes your esophagus, stomach, and intestines, and contains bacteria, viruses, fungi, and other microbes. The gut microbiome is home to trillions of bacteria, many of which produce neurotransmitters. These neurotransmitters play a role in regulating mood, anxiety, and pain.

The gut microbiome has a complex relationship with the nervous system. Emerging research suggests that it can strongly influence various aspects of your nervous system function, leading to stress and anxiety, and may contribute to the development or progression of neurological conditions, including Parkinson's disease, multiple sclerosis (MS), and Alzheimer's disease.[10] Studies have shown that changes in the gut microbiota composition can influence neuroinflammation, blood–brain barrier integrity, and the production of metabolites that can affect neuronal function and health.

The gut microbiome communicates with the brain through the *vagus nerve*. This is the longest of the twelve cranial nerves that connects to the brain stem and to many organs in the chest and abdomen, including the heart, lungs, stomach, intestines, and liver. It also plays a role in regulating heart rate, breathing, digestion, and other bodily functions. The vagus nerve is sometimes called the wandering nerve because it branches out to so many different organs. It is responsible for sending signals back and forth between the brain and the body and its roles include slowing down the heart rate; controlling the diaphragm; regulating the immune system; modulating pain; regulating mood and anxiety; stimulating the release of digestive juices; and helping to move food through the digestive tract.

The signals that your gut microbiome sends can also influence brain function, and vice versa. The gut produces and regulates the microbiome and produces and regulates neurotransmitters, which are the chemical messengers that facilitate communication between nerve cells in the brain. For example, certain gut microbes can produce neurotransmitters such as serotonin, dopamine, and gamma-aminobutyric acid (GABA), which are crucial for regulating mood, behavior, and cognition.

Your gut microbiome also interacts with your immune system, influencing its development and function. Your immune system consists of your thymus gland, bone marrow, lymph nodes and vessels, spleen, and skin. Your gut microbiome helps to educate and train the immune system, ensuring a proper response to anything that might cause disease, while maintaining tolerance to harmless substances. Dysregulation of the gut-microbiome–immune-system interaction can contribute to neuroinflammation and neurological disorders.

Imbalances or disturbances in the gut microbiome can also trigger an inflammatory response in the gut. This response can release various molecules and immune cells that can travel to the brain, leading to neuroinflammation.

Chronic neuroinflammation has been linked to neurodegen-erative diseases, mood disorders, and cognitive impairments.

In addition, your gut microbiome can influence your body's response to stress. It communicates with the stress-response system, including the hypothalamic-pituitary-adrenal (HPA) axis, which regulates the release of stress hormones such as cortisol. Disturbances in the gut microbiome can affect stress hormone levels, potentially impacting on mood, anxiety, and resilience to stress.

While research in this field is still evolving, evidence suggests that maintaining a healthy and diverse gut micro-biome through a balanced diet, regular exercise, adequate sleep, and stress management can positively influence your nervous system and promote overall well-being.

What you eat will affect not only your weight, but also the condition of your skin and hair and the good function-ing of your organs and nervous system.

Nourish with nature

Eating a range of natural foods is important for nourish-ing your nervous system, but so is your environment. Being in nature is a great way to soothe your nervous system and improve your overall health. Nature profoundly impacts the nervous system, offering numerous benefits for your men-tal and emotional well-being. Spending time in nature has been shown to reduce stress levels. Its calming effect helps to lower cortisol, a stress hormone, and promotes relaxation. This can decrease anxiety, improve mood, and enhance over-all well-being, positively impacting on your nervous system. But how does it do this?

If you remember from Chapter 5, our ancestors were hunter-gatherers, and it was critical to their survival that they could differentiate between the color of berries against the background of green foliage. We can still perceive the color green with the most ease because of how light reaches our eyes; the human eye translates waves of light into color.

The retinas in our eyes can detect light between wavelengths of 400 and 700 nanometers, a range known as the "visible spectrum." Each primary color corresponds to a different wavelength. The color red has the highest wavelength, blue has the lowest, whereas green is right in the middle of the spectrum. This is the wavelength where our perception is at its best. Blue and red light waves are enhanced and better perceived with the help of green waves, because green resides in the middle.

Being surrounded by green spaces might even help you to live longer. A 2016 study found that living in or near green areas was linked with longer life expectancy and improved mental health in women.[11] The data revealed that participants who lived in the greenest areas had a 12 percent lower death rate than women in the least-green areas. With more green space, the study authors said, came more opportunities to socialize outdoors. Additionally, the natural settings were more beneficial to mental health than more urban spaces.

Nature provides a respite from the constant stimuli and demands of our modern, technology-driven lives. Being in natural environments shifts our attention from directed, focused attention to more effortless "soft fascination"—this is a term that I use to mean not being focused on anything at all, just allowing your eyes to gently take in your surroundings. Restoring your attentional resources can improve cognitive performance, concentration, and mental clarity. Spending time in nature helps to alleviate mental fatigue and restore cognitive resources.

Engaging our senses in nature—such as feeling the texture of leaves, listening to birdsong or breathing in the fresh air—can ground us in the present moment and foster a sense of embodiment. The peacefulness, beauty, and serenity of natural settings positively influence mood, promoting feelings of happiness, calmness, and contentment. Nature also offers opportunities for physical activity and socializing with others, which can boost endorphin levels and enhance mood.

Nature has a multidimensional influence on the nervous system, encompassing stress reduction, attention restoration, mood enhancement, mindfulness, cognitive restoration, autonomic balance, and physical health benefits. Exposure to nature can also rebalance your nervous system. Spending time in nature activates the parasympathetic nervous system, or the rest, repair, and digest response, which promotes relaxation, digestion, and restoration.

Awe—or "wonderment"—is a complex emotional state characterized by a combination of astonishment, reverence, and a sense of vastness or transcendence. It typically arises in response to encountering something that is perceived as extraordinary, remarkable, or awe-inspiring. Awe can be triggered by various stimuli, such as witnessing natural wonders or contemplating the vastness of the universe, or by experiencing profound artistic or cultural expressions.

This is why stepping away from the grind of your day-to-day existence is so important. In awe-inspiring moments, people often feel a sense of humility, wonder and connectedness to something larger than themselves. The experience of awe can involve a shift in attention away from personal concerns and a heightened perception of the present moment. It may evoke feelings of admiration, inspiration, and a sense of being part of something bigger than yourself and your problems, which can lead to positive emotions, expansive thoughts, and a broadened perspective. I feel in a state of expansion when I am looking at art, listening to music or immersed in culture, listening to a clever podcast, watching a cinematic film, engaging in good conversation, watching the ebb and flow of the sea, and taking long walks in nature.

While awe is a subjective experience, researchers have explored its psychological, cognitive, and physiological dimensions to understand how it impacts well-being, cognitive processes, social behavior, and human experience. One study explored the relationship between awe and well-being.[12] The researchers found that individuals who reported experiencing more awe daily had higher levels of positive emotions, greater life satisfaction, and a lower tendency toward materialistic values. Awe was also associated with increased positive social behaviors and a sense of connection to others.

Overall, nature's impact on the brain encompasses stress reduction, attention restoration, mood enhancement, cognitive benefits, brain plasticity, mental-health support, physical-activity benefits, and opportunities for mindfulness and restoration. Incorporating regular nature experiences into your routine can have profound positive effects on brain health and overall well-being.

Case study: Natalie

Natalie came to me because she was unhappy. She was over-weight, which affected her health. She suffered from breathing issues and had severe bouts of depression. She had been in ther-apy for much of her adult life to overcome the effects of an unsafe childhood. Natalie had come a long way with therapy.

She lived in England but worked from home for a technol-ogy company in the US, meaning that her working hours were extended beyond a typical British working day. She went to bed at 1 a.m. as she liked to unwind by binge-watching her favorite TV shows. She existed on home deliveries. She didn't go outside very much. She rarely saw anyone in real life. She came to me because her current therapist suggested that Natalie should accompany her talking therapy with a body-based approach.

Natalie had unwittingly eliminated from her life all the ele-ments that we need for our nervous system to function well: living according to her circadian rhythm, moving every day, eating a diverse range of plants, recalibrating from micro-stressors throughout the day, breathing slowly to calm her system, having a community to support her, as well as keeping to a regular sleep pattern. I started by teaching Natalie movements to incorporate into her daily routine. She had a tense body, so I helped her to sense where she held her tension, and I showed her how to let that go. She had a pronounced forward-folding pattern; her head was forward of her shoulders and her shoulders rolled forward, contributing to her breathing issues. We worked on her breathing with movement, and she started to incorporate this into breaks from her screen.

Once Natalie gained control over her breathing and stress levels, I recommended a nutritionist to teach her how to cook and prepare tasty and nutritious meals. I also recommended a personal trainer that I knew, who worked with people with similar issues. This encouraged her to get out a few times a week and build a supportive community around her. It took a while, but over time Natalie understood the link between movement, food, sleep, and her mood. Working with her was a privilege, because she was committed and responded to the changes well. She lost weight and, more importantly, she gained a sociable and more meaningful life. She was able to manage her bouts of depression and stop a low mood from turning into anything more damaging.

Harnessing food and nature to soothe your nervous system

Now that you know how nature and nourishment affect your nervous system, you can make small changes toward making it function optimally. You could try to get outside as soon as you wake up, to signal to your circadian rhythm by getting light into your eyes. Incorporating movement outside is a powerful habit, as it combines two essential practices. Remember not to stare into the sun, as just being in the light without sunglasses is enough to wake up your system. Get out at dusk to attune your eyes to the fading light, too, which will prepare you for sleep.

Take a break from your desk often and, if you can, go outside and let your gaze soften. Regular breaks outside will soothe your brain. Get into the habit of leaving your phone at home on walks or switching it off. Try to avoid filling up all your spare time with mindless scrolling, as it stimulates your brain.

Eat unprocessed foods—ideally make your own meals—so that you know what ingredients you are eating. There are many good nutritionists to follow, so that you can find tasty recipes that include a wide range of plant-based foods.

Outdoors lesson

Try this lesson, which combines nervous-system soothing via your eyes with being outdoors:

1 If you can, sit outside in a place surrounded by greenery, where you can look out onto a horizon. You could also sit by a window, so that you can look out onto your garden or overlook a park.

2 Sit up on your sit bones, with your feet on the floor. Let your spine be long. Let your shoulders gently glide down, away from your ears. Close your eyes.

3 Take a slow inhale and a slow exhale. This is one breath. Repeat it twice more, so that you breathe in and out for three breaths. Slowly open your eyes.

4 Now take one hand about an arm's length away from you. Let your elbow be soft and hold your index finger up.

5 Allow your eyes to gently focus on your index finger. Carry on breathing at the slow pace.

6 As you do that, slowly let the index finger come toward you until it is approximately 6 inches away from your nose. As you breathe out, let your finger travel away from your nose, back to its original position. Keep your eyes with a gentle gaze on your index finger. Repeat this three times in total.

7 When you have completed three breaths while
   moving your finger, let your hand come down.
8 Let your eyes gently focus on the horizon. Notice
   how your eye muscles relax and your gaze softens.
   Feel how your face softens.
9 Breathe in and out for three breaths here.
10 Now let your eyes close and start the cycle again,
   inhaling and exhaling for three breaths. Complete
   three cycles and then let it go. Let your eyes be soft
   and, without moving your head or rolling your
   eyes, imagine that you are expanding your vision
   upward, downward, to the left and to the right.
   Let that go and let your gaze be soft and notice how
   you feel.

What you have learned in this chapter

- The food you eat will influence the quality of your
  nervous system. They will also influence your
  emotional mood. Include a diverse range of thirty
  plants in your weekly diet.
- Eat to keep your brain healthy by adding natural,
  unprocessed foods into your diet.
- Stay away from UPFs.
- Get outdoors as much as possible, especially first
  thing in the morning, at lunchtime, for a break and
  at dusk.
- Give yourself the opportunity to feel wonderment—
  it will get you out of your head and into the world.

We are going to look at connection in the next chapter:

connection to ourselves, to others and to our environment. But first, get outside and enjoy looking at the world with a soft gaze, and leave your phone in your pocket on silent.

8

Connect

In the end, these things matter most: How well did you
love? How fully did you live? How deeply did you let go?
Jack Kornfield, *Buddha's Little Instruction Book*[1]

A few years ago I moved from London, where I was born and
brought up, to a seaside town on the south coast of the UK.
I wanted more room, a garden, and a daily walk to the sea to
let my thoughts wander while gazing at the horizon. Once I
arrived, all those elements immediately gave me the sense of
relief and peace I had been craving.

What the move showed me that I hadn't realized, however,
was that I had also been yearning for a sense of community.
In west London I had lived in the same apartment for twenty
years. The apartments around me were generally owned by
landlords who were renting their spaces out, meaning that the
residents were transient. I have always been wary of getting
too close to people around me, as the anonymity permitted by
London life was something I enjoyed. Growing up, I lived in
one part of town, went out in another part, worked in clubs,
bars, and shops all over, and later grew my business around my
studios in central London. I had different friend groups all over
the city. I loved that freedom—the ability to shift and change

shape over the years, when forming an identity beyond my immediate vicinity and home. I didn't want the responsibility of maintaining many relationships with other people.

I prided myself on being self-sufficient because, in cities, you need to have an air of toughness to forge ahead. No eye contact on public transport or on the streets, as that can get you into a confrontation. Also, connecting with so many people on a single journey is exhausting, so you plug in your headphones and disengage. You learn to weave expertly around crowds of people without touching anyone, to get from A to B. In cities the game is one of avoidance. In smaller places, people smile at you or wish you good morning and take the time to stop and chat. At this time in my life I am in the right headspace to enjoy and cherish this level of connection with others.

The British anthropologist Robin Dunbar became convinced that there is a ratio between brain sizes and social group sizes, through a study of nonhuman primates. He concluded that the size of the part of the brain associated with cognition and language is linked to the size of a cohesive social group. Your brain evolved by moving you around your environment and adapting to survive in large and complex groups. Dunbar's number is the maximum number of other humans we can have a meaningful relationship with: that number is 150 contacts.

Your experiences are interwoven with the lives of others. To function well, you need three types of connections: to be in a relationship with yourself, to be in a relationship with others and to be in a relationship with the environment around you. The more we move away from these fundamental needs, the more ill at ease we tend to feel.

Connection to others

We have already discovered in Chapter 4, on touch, that babies have a strong attachment to their caregivers, and this relationship is critical to influencing how the brain develops. The relationship between the mother and the newborn starts in the embryo before birth. A newborn will prefer their mother's voice to anyone else's as they will have heard her voice in the womb. When the caregiver responds warmly and kindly to their baby, the interpersonal to–ing and fro–ing of tender experiences between the baby and her mother help the baby's brain develop. Attachment is an essential requirement of every human being. Without attachment to their caregiver, the human child cannot survive. You could also call attachment "love."

In collaborative hunter-gatherer societies in the past, children were always in nature with their parents, and they had many adults around them who acted as parent figures. The infant's brain learns to self-regulate with the mature adult brain. In contrast, in our modern Western communities, families usually live in small groups of two parents and their children, where women still bear the brunt of childcare and housework. Bringing up babies in a traditional nuclear family puts a great deal of stress on the family, with the father out at work and the mother often at home in isolation, looking after a newborn who is wholly dependent on her. Bringing up children in communities with multigenerational support was how we socially organized before we moved to cities, away from family and support. Mothers need support to repair and rest after the birth, and to benefit from the wisdom of elders who have given birth and raised families before them. We evolved to live in tribes, working in communities and with cooperation. Now that we have left our tribes, life often feels challenging.

While I'm not suggesting that we revert to those times, there is definitely something to learn from what we have lost— namely, the comfort of belonging to an intergenerational community that supports and nurtures those within it.

In our modern industrialized cultures we have normalized the physical and mental load placed on the mother by her taking full responsibility for food, entertainment, love, and the emotional regulation of her children, which is neither healthy nor sustainable. What does it teach our daughters and our sons? I remember, as a child, seeing the pressure that my mother was under and concluding that it was not for me. Motherhood without support appeared too stressful and thankless. I have many friends who felt the same, and my friends with children have confessed to me of feeling shell-shocked at how their needs are pushed out to the edges.

If we revisit the Romanian orphans, it was shown that those who had no contact with their caregivers beyond being fed and changed went on to suffer psychological effects that lasted a lifetime. Each child's outcome depended on when they were eventually adopted. If it was before the age of six months, the child would show normal development and an average IQ, but after that formative period the child usually found it difficult to have emotional bonds with others and scored a low IQ. A baby's brain is not fully formed at birth. Its development needs to be shaped by experience.

Connection to others and the wider world is as critical to your well-being as self-practice to regulate your nervous system. If you live with other people, you all co-regulate each other's nervous systems.

We each have a number of networks in our brain that generate social cognition—the information that we store and process about people around us. We have the amygdala network, which detects and processes key stimuli that attract our attention, such as our partner's voice, as opposed to that of a passing stranger. The mentalizing networks of our brain are activated when we think about people's feelings. The empathy network is activated when we think about other people's internal states. The motor cortex is involved when we think about other people's actions, including their emotional expressions and movements. Co-regulation is the process of regulatory support within our relationships enabled by these four networks working together.

Emotional co-regulation is a dynamic and reciprocal process and refers to how people mutually influence and modulate each other's emotional states in social interactions. It involves synchronizing emotions, non-verbal cues, and empathic responses between individuals, which contribute to regulating and maintaining emotional well-being. Emotional co-regulation is critical in fostering emotional connection and support; it means that human life is social life, and human connection works better face-to-face. Loneliness is often the first step toward emotional distress. Where did we learn the idea that being self-sufficient would be the most successful way to progress?

Love or loneliness profoundly affect your physical and mental state.

Connection to yourself

Have you heard of your "lizard brain"? It's the name for

the part of your brain that takes hold when you allow your instincts to overrule your decision-making. It is said that it was inherited from our reptilian past, before we evolved into human beings.

The concept of the "triune brain" was posited in the 1960s and suggested there are three layers to your brain, each emerging through evolution.[2] The first and deepest layer is the lizard brain, which functions purely on instinct. Your mammalian brain envelops the lizard brain and is the limbic system controlled by your emotions. The outer layer is the human brain, which rationalizes and reasons. The theory was that brain evolution is the reason we are in a relentless internal fight between our emotions and our rational brain. Except that this is not true, and this theory of the evolution of the human brain has since been generally discredited.

It is incredibly empowering to know that you are not at the mercy of an older part of your brain that you have to keep in check, using up your valuable resources. You are fully responsible for how you respond to events in your life. You will have learned behaviors, but you can replace them with newer ways to be. I have done it myself, and so have many of my clients.

An example of this that you might be familiar with is the rolling inner dialogue that tells you that you don't have enough money, you look old, fat, or too thin or aren't good enough. Compared to your friends and family, you aren't very successful. This inner dialogue never stops, generally spinning the same story about how worthless you are. Trying to bat away your internal dialogue is exhausting and sours your mood. And yet you give it your attention. But to replace this dialogue, you could try several things in order to minimize it. You could give your inner dialogue a name (someone whose opinion you don't value) or you could give it a funny high-pitched voice. Now that you don't identify the voice as yours, you can tell it to shut up. Just as you would if someone said those same mean things to you, you can also remind yourself of all the brilliant and courageous things you have achieved. Where you send your attention is where you send your energy. It is essential to pay attention to *what* you pay attention to.

Where you send your attention is something that you are very much in control of. For example, our culture is full of details about things we didn't think we were interested in. Yet we suddenly remember these most mundane details because they are mentioned everywhere. How much do you know about Jennifer Aniston? You know, Rachel with the much-copied hairstyle in the sitcom *Friends*? You might know that she is deemed unlucky in love, is very rich, has beautiful homes, loves yoga, has an enviable body, and rocks a bikini in her mid-fifties. You know this because the media aimed at women has pushed this information out into the world, so much so that there is a Jennifer Aniston neuron. This neuron activates whenever we see another story about her love life, body, lifestyle, or hair. The neuron is in a different place in different people, but the volume of information and the images of her have trained your brain to pull together concepts that build up a picture of Jennifer Aniston. With the rise of social media, which is more relentless in serving up information than traditional media, you don't have to go out and buy information. One minute you look at your friend's vacation snaps on her Instagram page; the next you get sucked into a vortex of disparate information. From pop culture to abandoned dogs, our attention is constantly under attack. I would even argue that your attention is your most valuable commodity.

Social media has hugely influenced how we communicate, engage, learn, and share information with the world. There were 246 million active social media users in the US as of 2023, representing roughly 72.5 percent of the American population. Facebook remains the most popular social media platform in the US, with around 177.5 million monthly active users as of 2023. While Facebook reigns supreme in user numbers, it's actually not the platform where US users spend the most time. That title belongs to YouTube, with an average daily usage of forty-six minutes per user in 2023.[3,4] The most popular way to access content is through mobile devices, meaning that you can access anything wherever you are. Social media has also changed the way your brain functions. According to recent data, the average person spends six hours and thirty-seven minutes on screen time per day across different platforms and devices. That equates to 44 percent of their waking hours. And one in five smartphone users spend three hours and forty-six minutes on their phones every day. Since 2013, global daily screen time has increased by eighteen minutes.[5]

Your brain is constantly being stimulated, and your neurons are firing throughout the day, which changes your brain's neurological structure. Your attention is seriously under attack. We looked at how the brain maps the body in Chapter 1. This is where regions of the cortex (the brain's outer layer of nerve-cell tissue) contain "maps" of the body's surface—particularly the motor cortex, which plans and creates motor contractions in your muscles; and the sensory cortex, which processes and rationalizes the information gathered by your senses. These maps differ for every individual, and change according to their life experiences. Your sensory and motor maps will depend on your habits. A concert pianist will have a different mapping of their hands from your own, dictated by how they use their hands and fingers. This is called neuroplasticity, and is the ability to change your brain over a lifetime.

When using the different social-media platforms, you view endless videos that run into each other, competing for your attention with textual overlays, ads, pop-ups, captions, comments, and likes. While processing this barrage of information, your concentration gets displaced across multiple incoming information streams. Your brain is now in perpetual multitasking mode, shortening your ability to pay attention and focus. Researchers believe that over time this shrinks the parts of the brain associated with keeping your concentration on one thing, making it harder for you to ignore distraction and leading to poorer cognitive performance. If your attention is constantly fragmented in this way, you are training your brain to be easily distracted. Controlling what you pay attention to can be your superpower.

The more you use social media to record and share your experiences, the more at risk you are of diminishing your actual memory of the experience. Social media affects your transactive memory: your ability to process information and store the memory. Social media is designed to be addictive and regulates your social and emotional responses. Regular users under thirty often compare themselves unfavorably to their social-media group. Likes and positive comments create a reward pathway in your brain and, conversely, the lack of positive comments or likes can make you feel anxious, sad, or depressed.

While self-comparison doesn't only exist on social media, you go through emotional processing much faster as you scroll down a screen than you do in real life. Studies have shown that positive and negative interactions online can also shape your behavior offline. You can see this in the hyper-real self-representation that is so common now, such as contoured makeup, which looks good on camera but is masklike in real life. Young children nowadays have a selfie-face they put on as soon as a camera points at them. Not allowing yourself to be fully yourself perpetuates the comparison cycle and leads to dissatisfaction with your real life, and to feelings of never being good enough.

Case study: Carly

Carly came to see me with chronic anxiety. Her public-facing job as a content creator meant she was always thinking about work. She had been successful for years, working with incredible brands around the world, but it took a toll on her well-being. She often felt anxious about her clients, and she found it hard to get to sleep as she had schedules and deadlines going around in her head. She tended to ruminate on the comments on her posts. She told me how, in her line of work, you can so quickly be out of step with the public mood.

Carly was drawn to fast action, big experiences, and doing. Nothing in her life seemed to be small, contemplative, or allowing her to be quiet. We worked together to find accessible practices that would allow her to self-reflect. Carly's body had been communicating to her through tightening, bracing, and clenching her jaw, but she paid this no attention. Over time this habit of tightening turned into a recurring shoulder injury, jaw aches, and, later, problems with her breathing, so that she sometimes had to gasp for breath.

When your life is fast, it can be challenging to be still, so I guided her through practices that allowed her to move slowly and rhythmically to soothe her noisy brain and listen in. Carly now has a library of bespoke, on-the-go practices at her fingertips that she can perform as she travels worldwide. She has morning, end-of-the-day and in-the-moment practices to help her deal with her feelings in real time, so she is no longer trying to push them away to get on with work. She was so used to feeling uncomfortable that she didn't know how else to be, but she now understands what it feels like to be comfortable in her body and can take the necessary steps to move into it. She has also carved out certain times in the day when she is online and other times when she can focus on creating content. She also makes sure that she has at least a day every week when she is not working.

Her partner is happier, as he didn't feel Carly was ever present with him. She can regulate her emotions to interrupt the sensations of anxiety. She no longer grinds her teeth, and her sleep is much improved.

We are so used to being connected online that it is the new normal to see couples or families eating in restaurants, each in their own separate world, focused on their screens instead of on each other. My puppy paws my phone out of my hand if he senses that I'm not paying him attention, and young children know when your attention has drifted away from them. I once met a tech entrepreneur who told me that his toddler used to swipe his face, expecting to be able to change his father's facial expression.

Your behavior influences the behavior of everyone around you. Being fully present is increasingly essential for you and the people you share your life with.

How to pay attention

Limiting distractions—such as social media, which eats up your attention—is the first step toward being fully present. I have built-in practices throughout my day to limit my phone use. I switch it off at night until my check-in time the next day, usually at 11 a.m. Limiting your screen time to thirty to forty-five minutes a day and having a designated time to use the apps is a much healthier way to approach social media, and allows your brain to focus on one thing at a time. Making an appointment to check in with your phone means that you control it, and not the other way around.

I don't regularly watch much TV—I didn't have a television for most of my adult life. I don't watch or listen to the news every day. I need peace and contemplation to think, plan and just be. I listen to podcasts that give me something to think about, I listen to music, I go to the movies and I like to read. I function better when my attention isn't being bombarded.

Once you have the space to do so, being able to pay attention prevents your brain from being overloaded with information. Your brain is bombarded with millions of bits of information per second, gathered from your senses. Specific neurons process all this information, but it would be impossible for your brain to look at each piece in detail. This is why your brain has a series of attention filters that perform selective processing by deciding what information is essential and allocating resources accordingly. Sifting through relevant information is fundamental to learning.

When you actively pay attention to certain information, it can have a cascading effect on the rest of your brain. The act of paying attention involves a selection process where specific neural networks become more active while others are suppressed. This is known as "selective attention." When the neurons responsible for paying attention become sensitive to the information you deem important, they enhance the processing of that information. This heightened activity leads to increased neural firing and to communication within the selected networks. At the same time, other competing or irrelevant neural networks are inhibited or suppressed, reducing their influence on cognition and perception. It has been shown that *how* you pay attention will change the shape of your brain, taking you from hypervigilance to a state of feeling calm and considered.

In one study researchers investigated the effects of learning a new skill—juggling—on the participants' brain structure.[6] Using magnetic resonance imaging (MRI), they found that after three months of intense juggling training, there was an increase in gray-matter volume in the mid-temporal area associated with visual motion-processing. These structural changes indicated neuroplasticity: the brain's ability to adapt in response to experience. What this tells us is that where once it was thought that your brain was hardwired as an adult and you were formed for life, you actually have the ability to alter how you respond to things; or, to put it another way, to change your idea of who you are.

Another way to sharpen your attention skills is through mindfulness meditation, which has become increasingly popular in recent years and comes from Buddhist disciplines that involve moment-to-moment awareness through contemplative practice. Long-term meditation practice has been shown to increase your resilience to stress as well as your compassion. It can undoubtedly improve mental health, although research shows that other practices, such as exercise and therapy, are just as successful.[7] This is good news for those of you who haven't resonated with meditation; don't worry, you can try another practice that enables you to be contemplative. A few of my neurodivergent clients, those with deep-held trauma, and Parkinson's clients come to mind. I give them rocking and rolling movements with breathwork instead, and it works just as well to soothe their minds.

Meditation comes in many forms, from simply focusing on your breathing or scanning your body, to more complex activities, such as observing your thoughts or focusing on an object. The common thread throughout meditation and awareness practices is that you first focus on your breathing. Throughout the practice you notice when your mind wanders, and when it does—it *always* does—you bring your attention back to the present moment. Knowing these two things is helpful because you can practice wherever you are, with few rules to follow.

However, many of my clients feel frustrated that they cannot meditate and it leaves them feeling like a failure—the recent popularity of the practice does not immediately mean that it's easy for everyone. Some people are highly attuned to their interoception, and some people have sharp auditory skills or even an ability to visualize. If you are not syncing with a particular form of meditation, it doesn't mean there is something wrong with you; it simply means that you are wired differently.

I prefer something other than rules-based practices; the stricter the rules, the less likely I am to practice regularly. Meditation was traditionally practiced in communities of men living in monasteries. They collectively cooked and cleaned; their lives were geared around meditation. Their lifestyles allowed for greater movement throughout their day, making sitting still more accessible.

This is crucial, because those of my clients who don't chime with meditation have minds that are too busy to enable them to sit still; for some people, sitting in stillness can overwhelm them. What works for one person might not work for someone else. And what once worked for you might not always work for you in every instance. My clients with different brain types have taught me how to adapt my teaching to suit them.

I prefer my contemplative practices to be mind-less, rather than mindful. To me, "mindfulness" always sounds as though it falls into the trap of doing more, whereas mindlessness is un-doing. I enjoy the not-thinking, the un-doing of my tightly wrapped mind as I garden or go for a walk among greenery, allowing my eyes to gaze softly. Or taking a train journey and staring out the window, watching the unfolding landscape, rather than scrolling through my phone. Allowing your brain to loosen its grip on thinking, assessing, and rating your actions and simply letting your mind wander is a powerful way to let your brain rest.

Have you noticed that you often find the solution to something that has been bothering you when you stop thinking about it? I have revelations on vacation that would never occur when I am sitting at my laptop trying to conjure up an outcome. Breaks from working, and sleeping between bouts of learning, enhance learning and reduce the likelihood of forgetting.

The brain learns in resting rather than in active thinking or doing mode, because of your *default mode network* (DMN). The DMN is a network of brain regions that are active when we are not focused on anything in particular. It is thought to be involved in self-reflection, introspection, and imagination.

When we are actively thinking or doing something, the DMN is suppressed. This is because the brain needs to focus on the task at hand. However, when we are resting, the DMN is allowed to become active.

There are a few different theories about why the brain learns in resting mode. One theory is that the DMN is responsible for creating a "mental map" of the world. This map is constantly being updated as we experience new things. When we are resting, the DMN is able to make sense of this information and store it in our long-term memory.

Another theory is that the DMN is involved in self-reflection and introspection. When we are resting, we have time to think about ourselves and our place in the world. This can help us to learn and grow as individuals.

Finally, the DMN may also be involved in imagination and creativity. When we are resting, we are free to let our minds wander. This can lead to new ideas and solutions to problems.

The science behind the brain's ability to learn in resting mode is still being studied. However, research suggests that it is an important part of the learning process.[8] When we give our brains time to rest, they are able to consolidate memories, make new connections between neurons and solve problems. This can lead to improved cognitive function and creativity—a surprising, inadvertent way of enhancing attention by temporarily seeming to lose it.

It must be noted, however, that you should rest your body

as well as your brain, as your ability to focus deliberately also depends on your sleep levels, which are crucial in achieving alertness. Research suggests that sleep helps learning and memory in two distinct ways. First, a sleep-deprived person cannot focus attention optimally and, therefore, cannot learn efficiently. Second, sleep has a role in memory consolidation, which is essential for learning new information. In a study, researchers investigated the effects of sleep deprivation on attentional networks using functional magnetic resonance imaging (fMRI). Participants underwent twenty-four hours of total sleep deprivation and then had fMRI scanning while performing attention-demanding tasks. The results showed that sleep deprivation led to significant impairments in attentional performance and to alterations in the functional connectivity and activation patterns within the brain's attentional networks.

Now that you understand how movement and activity soothe your brain and the rest of your nervous system, you can focus on finding practices that will help you to regulate your emotions rather than hinder your ability to practice on a regular basis.

How to change your nervous system

I have just talked a lot about paying attention and using mindfulness or mindlessness to hone your attention skills. Let's work with this idea, because paying attention is vital if you want to change your nervous system.

Why would you want to change your nervous system? As has played out in many of the case studies we've looked at, feelings of anxiousness, stress, and other negative emotions are formed by your past experiences and become the predictions that your nervous system draws on. You think you are feeling stress from overwork or an overflowing domestic task list, but it could also be true that your nervous system is producing uncomfortable feelings rooted in other things entirely, based on things that happened a long time ago. If this is the case and those feelings are disrupting your life, then you will need to change your nervous system to react differently. Neuroplasticity enables you to learn new things, to think differently, to minimize painful experiences and to adapt to whatever life brings.

Your vital functions, such as heart rate, digestion, and breathing, are hardwired to keep you alive. However, development plasticity happens from birth to twenty-five years old, as your nervous system becomes tailored to your experiences and discerns what you need to survive in your environment by learning to react in a certain way. This development plasticity enables your system to form new connections and to remove connections that you do not need. Positive and negative experiences are embedded at this stage.

However, when you are past the age of twenty-five, learning isn't as malleable or plastic as it is when you are young, and you have to actively engage in new learning in order to change your nervous system. You must learn differently if you want to teach your nervous system to react in different ways.

Having awareness of how you feel when something happens is the first step to changing your nervous system. When you are aware of a change that you want to make, specific chemicals get released in the brain that enable you to make those changes.

I'll give you an example. I used to bite my nails when I was younger, right down to the quick, until they bled and felt sore for days. There was something about biting my nails that gave me a distraction from my thoughts; it was an attempt at being embodied, although admittedly it wasn't a constructive way to feel in my body. As I grew into a young woman about town, with important jobs, I felt that my fingers belied my seemingly confident and in-charge persona. When gelled nails became widely available, I had a full manicure and allowed my real nails to grow underneath them. When I had the gels taken off, I had my own full nails and I stopped biting them. My nail-biting was a constant activity for twenty-five years, and it was rooted in my behavior. But I was able to stop it because I didn't want to bite my nails anymore, and in the interim I had learned other ways to soothe myself. However, in extreme situations, such as the death of my father and during the upheaval after the killing of George Floyd, I took to biting my nails again, as it was my default soothing system. As an adult, you don't unlearn habits, you simply replace them with new behaviors.

The nervous system changes when certain neurochemicals are released, allowing whichever neurons are active to strengthen or weaken their connections. If you think about what you are trying to learn and what you are trying to give up, the experience that you pay attention to will open neuroplasticity to that specific experience.

The chemical that floods your brain when you pay attention is the same chemical that is released during stress. Epinephrine is released in the brain when you are paying attention; it is called adrenaline when it is released from the adrenal glands, but it is the same chemical. Acetylcholine is another chemical in your brain that filters sensory input, and it acts as a spotlight and amplifies whatever you pay attention to. This chemical is released from another area of the brain. These chemicals combined will enable your nervous system to change. So you can see that the ability to pay attention to the way you feel has huge implications for your ability to soothe your nervous system.

Connection to your environment

Our culture lies to us. It sells us things we don't need by making us feel bad about ourselves and the world we have created. Many of us fill our lives by buying products and experiences to give it meaning and spend too little time on self-reflection. This turns us into passive consumers, trying to keep up with a version of ourselves that we want to project to the world. This disconnects us from who we are, which further disempowers us. But it is important to remember that you can also connect to your environment—socially, politically, economically, and ecologically.

It is no wonder that you feel frazzled and numb by buying more things, in the hope that it will soothe you. The thrill lasts for a short time and then you find yourself coveting the next item. Whole industries have sprung up around you not being *enough*. From the beauty industry through to fashion and lifestyle, it's all geared to keep you chasing something. Sometimes, when I felt lacking in life, I'd order expensive dresses and try them on with other items in my wardrobe. Then I sent them back, as the short-lived thrill was enough— it scratched the itch. The thrill was in having something *new* in my hands. I've since learned that there are so many other ways to soothe yourself *and* to do so in a way that is sustainable and nourishing.

Resisting this predominant message that you need to buy things to make you feel more alive will enable you to regain control of your well-being and your joy in life. Your actions matter. How you spend your money matters. Considering the broader picture of the impact of all that you buy is critical in flexing your connection muscle.

Who makes the dress that you bought for a party? The chances are it will be another woman on the other side of the world, who wasn't paid much and has no employment rights. There are 92 million tons of clothes-related waste each year worldwide, producing half a million tons of microplastics, and 57 percent of all discarded clothes end up in landfills; 93 percent of brands surveyed were not paying their garment workers a living wage.[9] The US is leading the ranking by revenue in the apparel market, recording $325 billion, followed by China.[10]

You might have heard of the concept of karma, which comes from yogic philosophy. "Karma" refers to the relationship between your actions and the consequences of your actions. Your actions leave a residue on the people you come into contact with, both in your community and in the wider world. It's about connecting to your surroundings and paying attention to how you live in the world.

Modern incarnations of spiritual practices have been subsumed by the culture that they once gave salvation to. Corporations co-opt mindfulness to keep their workforce productive; yoga teachers are sponsored by leggings manufacturers; spiritual baubles are a booming market. The psychic-services industry, including palmistry and tarot-card reading, is worth $2 billion a year in the US. Brands that enhance spirit and soul as their selling points are being manufactured to sell to Gen Z. Instead of tending to ourselves so that we might better tend to others, we seem to endlessly pursue self-improvement for its own sake.

I see clients who practiced yoga for many years. They meditated, ran, and worked out, but still felt disconnected— from themselves, their families, their work and from a purpose in life that is not necessarily connected to what they do, but to the values they hold. I have clients who have burned themselves out from working so much that somewhere along the way they forgot why they work so hard.

The more I work with people, the more I am convinced that connection is our first port of call when it comes to soothing the nervous system; that connection is first with ourselves, then with others, with our environment and with the ground beneath our feet.

Connection lesson

You will need to lie on a carpeted floor or a yoga mat; use a few thick blankets or throws if you're on a hard floor.

1 Lying down, let your arms and legs be long. If you can, lie with nothing underneath your head or knees, so that you can feel the back of your body on the floor on the same plane.

2 Notice how you feel on the floor. Take your awareness to the contact that your body makes with the floor. Let your mind's eye slowly wander down from the back of your head to your neck and down

to your shoulder blades, then sense the ribs that make contact with the floor. What do you feel next? Is it the back of your pelvis or perhaps the back of your thighs? Some of you will feel your calves as the next point of contact after your pelvis. And then you will feel your heels on the ground. How is the left part of your body different in terms of pressure on the floor from the right side of you?

3 Imagine if you were lying on memory foam: where would you sink in more? Where would you feel lighter? Breathe smoothly and slowly.

4 Sense the back of your head on the floor. And very gently, without disturbing your breathing, press the back of your head into the floor and then gently release the pressure. Think of the movement of a dimmer switch—it's a gradual movement rather than a sudden one. As if you are turning the volume up, and then turning it back down.

5 Now gradually let go of the additional pressure. Then repeat that action a few times, very slowly. Ensure you are comfortable and that it is easy.

6 Now let that go.

7 Then slowly go down your body to your heels, applying pressure in the same way with each body part, in this order:

- Skull a few times and then rest.
- Shoulder blades a few times and then rest.
- Space between the shoulder blades a few times and then rest.

- Ribs, which are already on the floor, a few times and then rest.
- Pelvis a few times and then rest.
- Calves a few times and then rest.
- Heels a few times and then rest.

8 Now reverse the sequence, traveling from your heels all the way up to your skull.

9 Rest.

10 And from your skull back down to your heels.

11 Rest.

12 Repeat this upward and downward pressure wave, but be sure to go slowly and to rest in between each part that you are pressing. Notice your breath throughout.

13 Let it go completely and notice how you make contact with the floor now, and how you are breathing. How do you feel? More connected? That was the idea.

What you have learned in this chapter

- As human beings, we are designed to connect: with ourselves, our community, and our environment.
- You can't control the chaos in the world, but you can control how you respond to things, by paying attention to what you give your attention to.
- You co-regulate your nervous system with those around you. Without others to regulate our emotions, our tolerance, patience, and empathy are reduced.

You have learned a lot about how your brain and body connect to work together as an interwoven system. Let's now review the principles of how to soothe your nervous system.

9

The Principles of The Soothe Program

You must understand the whole of life, not just one part
of it. That is why you must read, that is why you must
look at the skies, why you must sing, dance and write
poems, and suffer, and understand, for all that is life.

Krishnamurti, *Think on These Things*[1]

In the first eight chapters you have learned about your body
and how to sense it; you have discovered new senses and how
they work together to enable your brain to conjure up a fuller
picture of you and your environment. You have discovered
that breathing at a slower pace will change your emotions;
that touch goes deep; that movement is all about how we
move in the world; that rest is as important as action; that
when you nourish yourself, it makes you feel better. You have
learned that connection to yourself will help you connect to
others and to your environment.

Now that you have an overview of the workings of your
nervous system and an intimate idea of your relationship
with it, it is vital to understand the *why* as well as the *how*.
Read and reread these chapters, so that each time you take

in a little more information and you can sense the learning in your body—and try the lessons, either in order or as you prefer. All of them serve to teach you how your inner workings connect to your outside self.

To consolidate your learning, I am providing below the core principles of The Soothe Program, which serve as a summary and a crib sheet for all that we have covered together.

- **Adopt a bottom-up, top-down, outside-in approach**: cultivate the right conditions for physical and mental health through a comprehensive approach. Incorporate a bottom-up perspective by addressing physical signals from your body through movement, breathing, sleep, nutrition, and hormonal balance. Employ a top-down approach by exploring thoughts, emotions, and beliefs through practices such as meditation, conscious breathing, and self-reflection. Recognize the influence on your overall well-being of outside-in interactions, such as social support, therapeutic relationships, stress, life events, education, and environment.

- **Cultivate mind-body movement**: engage in movement practices that benefit both your brain and your body. Recognize the interconnectedness of physical and mental health, and prioritize movement that promotes curiosity and playfulness. Cultivate a harmonious relationship between your mind and your body through intentional movement. Your self-image comprises your physiology, sensations, emotions, thoughts, actions, and behaviors. How you move is all about how you move through life. Focus on organizing and aligning your bones in movement. Recognize the importance of proper alignment for optimal movement efficiency, stability, and injury prevention. Aligning your bones supports overall body functionality and well-being.

- **Learn experientially**: encourage experiential learning through sensing, imagination, curiosity, playfulness, movement, and tactile exploration. By actively engaging in self-exploration, we can deepen our understanding of ourselves, improve movement efficiency, and enhance our proprioceptive awareness.

- **Rest is radical:** embrace the significance of recovery and rest in your life. Understand that rest is essential and is a radical act of self-care. Incorporate periods of recovery, rest, and relaxation into your routine to restore energy, promote healing, and rejuvenate your mind and body. Utilize movement and breathing to soothe your brain. Understand that physical movement directly impacts your brain's functioning and your emotional well-being. Engage in movements that promote relaxation, stress reduction, and mental clarity. Acknowledge that transitions between activities are as important as the activities themselves. Prioritize moments of pause, recovery, and reorganization before action. You can approach each activity with intention and clarity by giving yourself time to pause, recover, and reset.

- **Metabolize your emotions**: allow your emotions to flow through movement. Understand that movement

can be a powerful tool for processing and releasing
emotions. When you are feeling stressed, choose
movement as an appropriate action to support
emotional and chemical release and overall well-
being. Address tensions in your body as they arise.
Develop awareness of physical tensions and release
them in the moment. Undoing tensions increases
freedom of movement, dynamic posture, and overall
well-being.

• **Adopt a strategy of expansion and retraction**: move
toward people, things, and challenges that makes
you expand, and away from anything that makes you
retract. Encourage elasticity and resilience in your
breathing, thinking, and movements. Recognize and
embrace the movements, people, and experiences
that bring growth and expansion in your life, while
consciously moving away from those that create
contraction and limitation.

These principles guide The Soothe Program, enabling you
to cultivate a compassionate relationship with yourself, to
optimize physical and mental health, and to promote overall
well-being.

Useful points of inquiry

• **Pay attention to your body**: what physical sensations
are you experiencing? Are you feeling tense, relaxed,
or do you not feel anything at all?
• **Notice your thoughts**: what are you thinking about?
Are your thoughts negative, positive, or neutral?

- **Consider the context**: what is happening in your life right now? Are you feeling stressed, happy, or something else?
- **Use specific language**: instead of saying, "I'm feeling stressed," try to say something like "I'm feeling anxious about my test results today and my mind is racing with anxious thoughts, which makes my breathing faster." This gives you a better idea of what action you can take to recover and reset.
- **Where in your body do you feel this emotion?**: tend to this part of your body first. Lying down on your back with your eyes closed is a good first step to soothe your system.
- **Be patient**: it takes time to find the right words to sense your feelings and better describe your emotions. Don't give up if you don't find them right away.

Part 2

The Soothe Program— Daily Practice

10

Waking Up

You wake up in the morning after a good night's sleep. Your brain is rested and recharged. You feel refreshed, rejuvenated and sharp. This is the perfect time to practice your 6:6 breathing (see page 100). A good way to incorporate a new habit into your life is to attach it to an existing one. My breathing practice happens before I brush my teeth. I sit up in bed and go straight into my breathing, before anything has the potential to distract me. I don't take my phone into the bedroom, to avoid the temptation of checking social media or any messages first thing in the morning. Instead I use a digital metronome to practice with.

Start your breathing practice with five minutes daily, and build up to twenty minutes a day over a few months. Consistency is crucial, as that is how you shift your nervous system's baseline. Breathing will enhance mental clarity and set the tone for the day ahead. You'll have energy for the day and will remain on an even keel, as breathing slowly will boost your mood.

The more you get used to practicing this pace of breathing in the morning, the easier it will be to incorporate it into a movement routine. The following joint mobilizations are quick and easy to remember in the morning and you can do it while practicing your breathing. If you can do it outside in your garden or a park, then you've ticked three critical practices to get you energized and prepared for your morning: breath, movement, and daylight.

Joint mobilization

1   Start in a comfortable standing position with your feet shoulder-width apart, knees slightly bent and arms relaxed by your sides. Close your eyes and take a few deep, slow breaths to center yourself.

2   Begin by gently shaking your body from head to toe, allowing any tension or stiffness to release. Shake out your arms, legs, and whole body for about thirty seconds to a minute.

3   Now, turn your attention to your ankles and feet. Take a step back with one leg, rest on the ball of the foot and gently rotate your ankle in a circular motion. Make sure you roll onto the front and sides of your toes and tuck the toes under—this ensures that you are also rolling through the toe joints. Perform five to ten rotations in each direction. Step that foot sit-bone distance apart from the standing foot. Repeat the same movement with the other foot.

4   Send your attention to your hips and knees. Stand with your feet hip-width apart and place your hands on your hips. Slowly rotate your hips in a circular motion, as if you are stirring a large pot with them. Perform five to ten rotations in each direction.

5   Now bend your knees slightly and gently bounce up and down without lifting the heels, as if you were on

a bouncy floor, allowing your body to relax and your joints to loosen. Perform this bouncing movement for about thirty seconds.

6 Bring your attention to your spine. Bend your knees a little. Place your hands on your lower back, with your fingers pointing toward your spine. Begin gently twisting your torso from one side to the other, letting your arms drop down and allowing them to swing naturally. Let the movement flow from your waist, keeping your feet grounded. Perform five to ten twists in each direction.

7 Take your focus to your neck and shoulders. Slowly roll your shoulders up to your ears, backward and downward in a circular motion, making gentle and smooth rotations. Repeat this movement five to ten times. Then reverse the direction and roll your shoulders forward, downward, backward, and upward the same number of times.

8 Now move to your wrists and hands. Extend your arms straight out in front of you, palms facing down. Make a gentle fist and slowly rotate your wrists in a circular motion, first in one direction and then the other. Perform five to ten rotations in each direction.

9 Now, with your knees slightly bent, take your arms up overhead and grab one forearm with the opposite hand and side-bend over to the opposite side. Let your ribs come together on the side you are bending toward, and let the spaces between your ribs on the other side open. Breathe into your waist and armpit for one breath. Come up and release the arms, then

swap over and repeat on the other side.

10 To finish, come back to whole-body shaking for thirty seconds and then stand still for a moment, take a few deep breaths and observe how your body feels. Notice any sensations of tingling, warmth, or releasing.

This routine will wake you up for the day ahead and transition you from lying down to a more active mode. Can you walk outside—perhaps some of the way to work or taking the children to school? Try to fit into your day as much walking outdoors as you can.

Break up your laptop work with eye breaks at least every twenty minutes, plus, ideally, whole-body breaks where possible. Try to look out of a window and let your eyes look to the far distance every twenty minutes. You can also warm your hands and cup your eyes, resting your hands on the sockets around the eyes. Keep your fingers and thumbs close to each other and let the warmth of your hands soften the muscles around your eyes.

Eye lesson

Familiarize yourself with this lesson before attempting it, because it needs to be done with your eyes closed.

1 Close your eyes and slowly roll your eyeballs in their sockets to the left, back to the center and a little to the right. Make it a small movement in each direction. Avoid stretching or pulling on the eyeballs. Imagine them as little plums, and as you

roll them, think about the front, sides and back of the rolling eyeball. Do they feel smooth all the way round? Is your left eyeball more responsive than your right one? Can you match the pace of your more responsive eyeball to the less responsive one?

2   Let your eyes rest in the middle. Slowly take your eyeballs to the top left of your eye sockets and then slowly down to the right in a diagonal line. Trace this line slowly a few times. Notice how easily both eyeballs can roll in this new direction. Let your eyes rest.

3   Now take both eyeballs to the top right of your socket and then to the bottom left, being careful not to stretch your eyes. Trace this line slowly and steadily a few times. If you go too fast or hard, your brain will not be able to listen to essential signals from your eyes, face, and the rest of your body. Let your eyes rest.

4   Slowly allow your eyeballs to trace a smooth figure eight on its side, crossing the figure eight over your nose. Start either on the left or the right, whichever you find most accessible, and begin by drawing a small figure eight, so that you are not stretching your eyeballs in any direction. The movement should be smooth and easy, and do you no harm. Rest your eyes. Don't forget to go the other way around the figure eight.

5   When you have finished, breathe and slowly blink your eyes open. Notice how you feel.

These eye movements might feel clunky to start with, but over time you will notice a smoother pattern of movement.

Keep it small, reduce your range and rest when you have lost your focus—and breathe.

In your seat

We sit a lot more than our ancestors did, which means it is crucial that we include movement into our periods of sitting still.

1 Sit up on your sit bones toward the front edge of your seat. Imagine that you are sitting on a clock face: twelve o'clock is forward, which means that six o'clock is behind you.

2 Using a small range of movement, roll your pelvis between twelve o'clock and six o'clock, letting your spine (including your head) follow the movement. In sitting, your nose will travel in the opposite direction to your pubic bones. When you roll to twelve o'clock, your nose travels upward; when you roll to six o'clock, your nose travels downward. Let your spine respond to your pelvis. You can match one part of your breath to one part of your movement.

3 You can now vary this by rolling your pelvis clockwise around the clock face. Let your hands rest on your lap, with your palms facing up. Notice how your ribs also roll around in a clockwise direction, and your breastbone lifts and sinks as it travels in a circle around the clock face. Let your spine be influenced by your rolling pelvis, so that you let the movement flow to your head, allowing it to roll too.

4 Rest and sit up on your sit bones, noticing how you

now have more sensation in your pelvis, lower back, ribs, shoulders, neck, and head.

5   Reverse the direction of the circle, so that you now take your pelvis in an anticlockwise direction.

6   Rest and notice how you feel.

The beauty of this movement is that you can simply practice the twelve to six o'clock action in your pelvis so that no one knows you are doing very much, or you can make a bigger circling movement if you are working from home. I encourage my clients not to mind appearing weird in public spaces. Caring deeply for yourself is a radical act of compassion, so you need to be fearless about grabbing opportunities for practice throughout your day.

11

Midday

You've been working and in the same position all morning, so it's time for a break from what you are doing. If you can, get out to walk in greenery, as this will let your brain and eyes rest but get your body moving. Try not to fill up your time with calls and scrolling; even better if you can leave your phone behind. Aim for at least a few hours a day without your phone. I have trained myself to check my phone and email at specific points throughout the day. This means that I can focus on deep work using intermittent resting, as laid out in Chapter 6.

Get your body moving for short bursts. This could include shaking, jiggling on the floor, or these arm swings:

Helicopter Arms

1 Take off your shoes and stand, resting into your feet, with your knees slightly bent.
2 Raise your arms up to the ceiling, without stretching at full range.
3 Choose your dominant arm and start to circle it backward, as if you are trying to draw a circle in

space—you can pick up the speed. Let your chest
and head move as they wish to.

4 Let the other arm circle in the opposite direction.
Allow the movement to travel through you; this
means that your torso, including your chest and
belly, will move to accommodate your arms circling
in opposite directions.

5 Let your arms come to rest and notice the liveliness
in your torso, arms, and fingers.

6 Reverse which arm circles backward and which one
forward.

Moving your arms in opposing circles is good for your brain,
will mobilize your chest, arms, and head, and will move you
out of your habitual patterns of movement.

Wall clock

1 Stand with your right side against a wall. If you can't
get to a wall, you can do this in space. Eventually
you will be drawing a circle with your arm, keeping
close to the wall. You will be turning your torso into
the wall when you need to take your arm behind you,
and back to face forward again—the movement
comes from your waist upward.

2 Let your arms dangle down and with your right
shoulder, right arm, and as much of your leg and
foot as is easily possible, make contact with the wall.
Imagine a clock face drawn on the wall: your head is at
twelve o'clock and your feet are at six o'clock. Forward
is nine o'clock and behind you is three o'clock.

3   Your right arm is the hour-hand: when it is by your
    side it is at six o'clock. Slowly slide your right arm
    up, with the back of your hand on the wall, to seven
    o'clock and back to six o'clock. When your arm
    moves away from six o'clock, press your right hip
    against the wall; when the arm comes back, move
    the hip to make space for the arm to return to its
    starting position.

4   Do this a few times. Move slowly and keep your arm
    and the back of your hand sliding against the wall,
    as the feedback is important for your brain.

5   Now slide it up to eight o'clock and back through
    seven and six o'clock. Do this a few times. Rest with
    your hand at six o'clock.

6   Now slide to nine o'clock and back through eight,
    seven, and six o'clock. Do this a few times. Rest with
    your hand at six o'clock.

7   Slide your arm up through seven, eight, and nine to
    ten o'clock and all the way back to six. Do this a few
    times. Rest with your hand at six o'clock.

8   Slide your arm up to eleven o'clock and all the way
    back to six. Do this a few times. Rest with your hand
    at six o'clock.

9   Slide your arm right up to twelve o'clock and all the
    way back to six. Do this a few times. Rest with your
    hand at six o'clock.

10 Slide your arm up to twelve o'clock and start to turn
    your hand so the palm faces the wall and allow the
    opening and turning of your chest toward the wall.
    The turning of your palm to the wall enables you to
    circle behind you to one o'clock and then turn onto

the back of the hand to come back through twelve
to six. Keep your arm long and reaching, but not
stretching. You want to feel your ribs opening, and
your torso turning will enable that to happen.

11 Keep your right side against the wall. Your pelvis
and knees should stay more or less forward, but
not rigid. The turning is coming from your waist
upward.

12 Slowly in this way, with your arm sliding against the
wall, turn your chest in toward the wall to find the
hours two, three, four, five, and six and all the way
round through nine to twelve again. You are now
drawing a big circle on the wall with your arm, by
allowing your chest and torso to soften and turn into
the wall.

13 When you have traveled around the clock face in a
clockwise direction a few times, let your arm dangle
down by your side and move away from the wall.
Notice how much space you now have in your right
arm, chest, back, neck, and side-body.

14 Go back to the wall and this time stand with your
left side against it and, slowly but surely, explore the
hours to three o'clock and then up to twelve o'clock,
and at some point turn your palm toward the wall
and start to enjoy the journey, hour by hour. Avoid
going too fast or jumping to a full circle straight
away. Be interested in the process of sliding your arm
to each hour and back again, and in how your chest,
armpit, torso, belly, waist, and ribs open and rotate
to accommodate the circling of your arm. Once you
are drawing a full circle in an anticlockwise direction

and have done it a few times, let your arm rest at six o'clock again and walk away from the wall.

15 Notice the openness, the length, the release, and the space. How do you feel with this new space?

Jaw, tongue, and mouth lesson

Your head, eyes, and neck get stuck in one position every time you assume your laptop pose. Your head is forward of your spine, your eyes are fixed on your screen, the back of your neck is contracted, and your shoulders rise up to your ears and stay there. You hold your breath. Let's unstick this position.

1 Come up to standing; ideally you should have no shoes on. Notice how you stand: do you slump downward? Where do you take the load? In your neck, lower back, knees? Is the weight on the big-toe part of your feet or on the little-toe side of your feet? Where do you feel tense or sore?

2 Check in and notice how your mouth feels. Are you clamping your jaw? Biting into your tongue?

3 Now sit down toward the front edge of your seat. Notice how you breathe and keep a steady inhale and exhale throughout this lesson.

4 Take your tongue to the front of your upper teeth— breathe easily here. Keep your lips lightly closed, but let your jaw open and move as it needs to. Slowly slide your tongue to the right until you arrive at the last tooth on your right upper jaw. Slide your tongue back to the middle. Repeat this action of sliding

your tongue from the middle to the last tooth on the right. Feel the surface of each tooth: let your tongue travel across every curve, gap, and bump.

5 Now rest your tongue and mouth. Notice how the right side of your mouth feels. How does your tongue feel? Your jaw?

6 Now take your tongue and rest it in the middle of the front bottom row of your teeth. Slide your tongue to the right until you get to the last tooth of the bottom row and then slide it back to the middle. Do this a few times, exploring every tooth on the bottom row from the middle to the right and back again. Your tongue should slide lightly, so that it can feel around the surface of each tooth.

7 Now rest your tongue and mouth. Notice how the right side of your mouth feels. Soak in the new sensations.

8 Take your tongue to the middle front upper teeth, and this time slide it to the last tooth on the upper right, then down to the last lower tooth on the right and across to the middle lower tooth, then back up to the upper-row middle tooth. Keep sliding your tongue in a clockwise direction, exploring the whole right side of your upper and lower teeth. When you have done this a few times, rest and then go round the other way.

9 Rest your tongue and jaw and notice what you sense.

10 Take your tongue and press it into your right cheek. Release it, then do it again a few times. Rest.

11 Now take your tongue into your right cheek and draw a circle around the inside of it in a clockwise

direction. It will look like you are rolling a gobstopper
in your mouth. Fully explore the inside of your right
cheek with your tongue. Rest your tongue, mouth,
and jaw. Reverse the direction of the circle.

12 Rest. Notice how you have space in the right side of
your mouth and how your jaw hangs effortlessly. Does
the right side of your face feel longer than the left side?

13 Now explore the right side of your mouth using your
tongue, including your upper and lower teeth, right
into the gaps between the last tooth and the inside
of your mouth, the inside of your upper and lower
lips. Use you tongue to get into all the nooks and
crannies of the right side of your mouth and teeth.

14 Rest. Notice that you now have space in your upper
palate, the back of your jaw and underneath your
jaw. Notice how the right side of your tongue feels
fuller, more tingly and livelier.

15 Come up to standing and notice how you feel
upright on the right side, as if you are lifting up
from the floor. How does the left side feel? A little
heavier, denser, and sunken?

16 Come back to sitting and explore the left side of
your upper and lower teeth, the inside of your cheek
and the left side of your mouth, using the same steps
as above. Rest in between each step.

17 When you have fully explored the left side of your
mouth, let your tongue go around the whole mouth
from left to right in a clockwise direction, and then
in an anticlockwise direction a few times.

18 Rest. Notice the space and tingly sensations in your
face, jaw, mouth, and tongue. Come up to standing

and notice how you feel yourself lifting up and away from the floor.

Once you learn this lesson, you can do it anywhere and in any position. I practice it every day while I am writing—it acts as a freshener and helps me to formulate my ideas. I also use this lesson before I am being interviewed for podcasts, as it stimulates my face and tongue in preparation for speaking and being on camera. It also helps to lift the jaw and exercise the facial muscles, which is another good reason to practice it often.

As well as formal practices, remember to soothe yourself if something comes up for you and makes you feel anxious or stressed. I call these "micro-soothe practices" to soothe you from the micro-stresses that happen in your day. Say you receive an email that makes you hold your breath—get up and shake it off. Or roll your shoulders, go outside, or move in some way. Remember that experiencing an intense feeling but taking no action leads to tense muscles, which will influence your mood. Make sure you move it out of your body.

Try this micro-soother with the wrists

1 Sit on your sit bones and loosely interlace your hands, then place them palms down on your belly.
2 Notice your breathing. Keeping your thumbs on your belly, roll your palms away from it—the little-finger side rolls up; it is a very small movement. You are creasing a little at your wrists as your knuckles roll toward you. As you exhale, release back to the starting position of having your little fingers on the belly.

3   Do this a few times. If you were being watched, no
    one would know that you are moving at all.
4   Rest from this. Notice how you feel.
5   Come back to this practice, but this time, as you
    inhale, also nod your chin up a little. Again, this is a
    tiny movement. As you exhale, release your chin. Do
    this a few times.
6   Now let that go, undo your hands and notice how
    you feel.

I realize that when you are working in an office with other
people, some of these practices may make you look strange,
but they will also make you feel calmer. And you are dealing with your feelings as they come up. You could go to the
bathroom or a meeting room; you could also teach these
lessons to your colleagues, set a timer throughout the day
and practice them together, helping to regulate each other.
The more you do them, the more you normalize deep care
for yourself.

12

Day's End

If you have been in the same position all day, now is the time to move. Walk part of the way home or, as soon as you get there, put on some music that you like to dance to and move, shaking out your arms and legs. Maybe even get everyone else in your house to join in—it's a joyous way to connect to each other after a day apart, which doesn't involve an inquisition. After you've moved your day out through your body, you will have richer conversations that don't focus on the problems you've encountered.

Wide-legs swing

You can also try this simple wide-stance swing:

1 Take a big, wide-legged stance and bend at your waist as if you are about to sit down on a high stool.
2 Imagine that you are holding a large boulder with both hands. Now imagine that you are throwing your boulder, first to the left and then to the right. Let your shoulder blades slide over your rib basket and let your opposite heel come up. You will bend both knees in the middle as you swing over to the

opposite side. Imagine the heaviness of the boulder; it requires you to bend in the middle and swing it to one side and then the other. The swing should feel flowing and freeing.

3 Do this six times from one side to the other and get into a rhythm.

Rolling with interlaced hands

Make some time after work, and before you run around, to get down on the floor. The lessons in this chapter will take you fifteen to twenty minutes and will help to recalibrate your nervous system before you get busy with your family and life. A well-organized person regulates those around them, which makes caring for yourself as important as caring for others.

Most of us are in "doing" mode most of the time, and we need to relearn how not to be. It is a state of being that is distinct from anticipating the next action, or even holding your breath. You want to be able to make these distinctions, so that you learn to feel again. This is where you have a choice: the choice lies in the quality of your actions, and you can exercise this by moving slowly, doing less, and being guided by how the action feels. Tuning in to the choices that you have will help you transition from your working day, and from a fixed state to a place where you are more curious—a place where you can meet your life exactly as it unfolds.

1 Come to lie down on the floor. Notice which parts of you yield easily and which parts of you feel tense and tight. Breathe into and out of your belly a few times.

2 Bend your knees and interlace your fingers loosely, placing the palms on your chest and keeping your elbows on the floor or weighted toward the floor.

3 Lift your right elbow just a little away from the floor and then place it down again, keeping your palms on your chest. The lifting of your elbow should feel easier and more comfortable each time. Rest before you try it again.

4 Notice the right side of your collarbone and how it moves. What happens in your right shoulder blade: does it move away from your spine or toward it? How does the movement differ from your left shoulder blade?

5 Now come to rest, letting your arms lie by your side and sliding one leg away and then the other. How do you contact the floor: is it different from at the start of the lesson?

6 Open your mouth and let your lower jaw drop away from your upper jaw, then slowly bring your lower jaw toward your upper jaw again. Do this a few times.

7 Let your lower jaw hang. Open your mouth and slide your jaw to the left and back. Make this a small, slow movement, and stop before you stretch or push. Think about moving from your jawbone, not from your lips or the skin on your face.

8 Now bend your knees, interlace your hands and place them on your chest, with an open mouth. Lift your right elbow at the same time as your lower jaw slides to the left, then bring your elbow down at the same time as your lower jaw slides back.

9 Rest when you come back to your starting position,

where your elbow is back on the floor and your jaw is in the center, with your mouth closed. Repeat this sequence a few times; it should feel easier and more comfortable each time.

10 Rest as you are.

11 Now leave your jaw alone and just lift and lower the right elbow. Is it different or easier?

12 Rest with your legs long and notice the space in your upper back on the right compared to the left.

13 With your legs long, clasp your hands and place them on your chest again. This time lift and lower your left elbow. How does it feel to switch to this side? Do it slowly and make the movement small in range, so that you can feel the transfer of weight with your contact on the floor, and do not disturb your breath.

14 Rest from this but stay as you are.

15 Now bend your knees and lift and lower your left elbow. Is this easier with bent knees? How does it feel easier on a sensation level? Try this a few times and listen in to the quality of your movement.

16 Rest from this.

17 Now let your lower jaw hang and, as you lift the left elbow, slide your jaw in the opposite direction and, as you lower your elbow, let your jaw slide back. Do this a few times, but in such a way that you can sense how you make this movement. How is your weight transferring on the floor?

18 Rest from this.

19 Now open your mouth, let your jaw hang a little, lift your right elbow, roll your head and eyes to the

left and slide your jaw to the left. Lower your right
elbow as you roll your head and eyes back and slide
your jaw to the center. Do this as if your jaw is
moving away from the center and coming back to it
in one movement. Repeat a few times.

20 Rest as you are.

21 Repeat this with your left elbow, letting your head
roll to the right and your jaw slide to the right. Lower
your left elbow and let everything come back to the
center. Try this a few times, allowing all the seemingly
different types of movement to work in harmony.

22 Rest with your legs long and your arms by your sides.

23 Bend your knees again and place your feet on the
floor. Interlace your fingers and rest your hands on
your chest. Lift your right elbow, rolling your head
and eyes to the left. Keeping your feet on the floor,
tilt your knees to the left and then bring everything
back to the center. Do this a few times.

24 Rest from this.

25 Practice the same sequence of events, but this
time also slowly rotate your palms away from you,
lengthen your arms and push your palms and arms
out diagonally into the air space on your left as you
roll onto your left side. Then rotate your palms back
and reverse the movement to come back to the floor,
with your knees bent and your palms back on your
chest. Do this in small increments until you roll onto
your left side. Think about how you will reverse this
sequence to return onto your back to the starting
position. Play with this movement a few times to
find the most comfortable and lazy way to do it.

26 Rest on your back, with your legs long and your arms by your side.

27 Repeat steps 23–25 a few times with your left elbow, rolling onto your right side.

28 Now rest completely, with your legs long and your arms long by your sides. Notice what imprint you make on the floor now: what parts of you contact the floor and how is it different from before? How is your breathing, and what parts of you accommodate your breath? How do you feel now?

29 From here, slowly open your eyes and bend your knees to roll over to one side and come up to sitting. You will find that your working day now feels distant and you can get on with your home life, with some headspace.

I start getting ready for bed at least an hour before I want to be in bed. As 10 p.m. is the time I aspire to be *in bed*, that means I need to start getting ready at 9 p.m. I lie on the floor just to rid myself of any tension, so that when I am in bed I can more easily fall asleep. I do this in my pajamas, after I have bathed, and just before I slip into bed. It doesn't take me long.

Walking the spine

1 Lie on the floor, letting your bones descend. Start to notice your breathing. Notice the shape that you make on the floor: if you were lying on memory foam, what sort of shape would you make?

2 Jiggle your body on the floor.

3 Let it go and notice how you feel much wider.

4 Bend both knees and place your feet on the floor. Let
   your arms lie by your side.

5 Slowly start to press your feet into the floor. Feel
   your pelvis get lighter, but don't lift it from the floor.
   Then gradually let go of this pressure, so that the
   pelvis weights back into the floor again. Do this a
   few times.

6 Now press just one foot into the floor and let your
   hip roll away from the floor; the same knee travels
   forward, not inward, as you release the pressure
   of this foot, let the hip roll back down. The hip is
   rolling away and back down to the floor; it is not
   lifting straight up and down.

7 Now press the other foot into the floor and let this
   hip roll away from the floor; let it come down as you
   release the pressure of the foot.

8 Alternate from foot to foot, so that you are rolling
   one side of the hip away and then the other. Now
   pick up the pace, so that it resembles the jiggling
   motion, but this time you are moving from side to
   side. Let your head roll in the same direction as your
   hip to begin with.

9 Rest from this.

10 Now do the whole movement again, but this time let
   your head roll in opposition to the hip. Do not force
   your head, but let it roll lazily on the floor. This
   movement releases the spine, pelvis, head, and your
   neck to prepare you for rest.

Get-ready-for-sleep breath

1. Lie on your back in bed with your lights dimmed. Breathe in and then let your breath go, taking the time you need for each breath.

2. Place your hands on your abdomen, with your thumbs on each side of your navel. Your thumbs should have space between them; softly let your fingers span out without stretching. It is as if you have a breathing sphere underneath your hands.

3. As you breathe in, your belly rises and expands into your hands, and as you exhale, your belly moves softly away from your hands. This is a soft breath. As you inhale, imagine the space between the thumb and index finger of each hand getting a little wider; as you exhale, this space gets narrower. It is as if your hands are moving in time with your breath. You are not making this happen—you are sensing it happening.

4. Now, as you exhale, imagine that you are bringing the thumb and index finger a tiny bit together, as if you are pinching the skin on your belly. It is a small and gentle movement. Stay in the realm of imagining that you are doing it, and now actively move them exactly as you imagined. If you were being watched, no one would know you were moving your thumb and index finger together.

5. Now rest from this activity, keeping your hands there and allowing them to follow the movement of your belly.

6. Take your hands away and rest. Notice how you breathe and where you breathe into.

7   Now take your hands onto the lower ribs on each
     side. Keep the space between your thumb and
     index finger. As you breathe in and out, notice the
     small movement from expanding to retracting the
     space between the thumb and index finger. On an
     inhale they move apart, and on an exhale they move
     together.
8   Now exaggerate this, with minimal movement
     between the thumb and index finger of each hand.
     As you exhale, bring these fingers toward each
     other; as you inhale, let them release. Let your exhale
     draw the thumb and index finger together in the
     gentlest of movements, and let your inhale gradually
     relax your hands. Do this a few times. The smaller
     your movements, the more deeply your system will
     relax.
9   Rest quietly, with your hands where they are.
10   Now let your hands move away and notice the
     movement of your ribs.
11   Place your hands just underneath your collarbones,
     with easy space between your fingers and index
     finger and thumb. Follow the same practice as above,
     repeating steps 7–10, but with hands under the
     collarbones.
12   Let your hands come down by your sides and notice
     the movement of your belly, ribs, and chest as you
     breathe in and out. Slowly let that go and enjoy a
     restful night of sleep.

13

Emotional Rescue

In the absence of social interaction that
feels safe . . . nobody can be expected to be
healthy, happy, or able to think right.

Stephen Porges, *Our Polyvagal World*

What to do when your routine goes out of the window? Clients often tell me that when they go away for work or for pleasure they stop practicing, because the new experience takes over. That is completely understandable, but the intention is that your soothing practices are an integrated part of your life so that, no matter where you are or what is required of you, you can still function at your optimum.

The first thing I do after a flight, or when I'm away from home, is to take my shoes off and place my feet on the earth. After being in the air or traveling, a grounding practice is what I need. When you are in the same position for a while, your muscles tense and you lose all the subtle sensation of your physical body, which affects how you move and will go on to influence your emotions and your thoughts.

Rolling through your spine

A good first step is to tune in to what you feel.

1   Come to lie down on the floor.
2   With your legs long and your arms by your sides,
    concentrate on your breath. Notice how your belly
    rises on the inhale and falls on the exhale. Where
    else can you feel your breath? Notice how the
    pressure on the floor changes with your breath.
3   In your imagination, run through the curves of
    your spine, from the back of your head through
    to your neck, your shoulder blades and the space
    between your shoulder blades, your ribs, lower back
    and pelvis. Travel up and down your spine in your
    imagination a few times.
4   Bend one knee at a time and place your feet on the
    floor. Notice how the curves of your spine change
    when you bend your knees, and how your weight
    transfers on the floor.
5   Keeping your pelvis on the floor, roll your tailbone
    away from the floor and release it (your tailbone isn't
    on the floor, but the direction of movement is away
    from the floor). Make this a small action of rolling
    your pelvis on the floor like a rolling pin. Do this
    a few times. You are looking for a smooth rolling
    action. Now let it go.
6   Roll your pelvis up until you are at the top of your
    sacrum—this is the bone in between your two pelvic
    halves at the back of you. Do this a few times,
    making this movement small and slow, so that you
    can sense how you roll the pelvis toward and away

from you. Rest and notice where your pelvis rolls
back into position.

7   Now roll your pelvis up to the top of the pelvic bone
and then let it roll back to rest. Do this a few times.
Which movement is more familiar to you? Rolling to
the top of your pelvis or rolling back again? Let it go
and rest.

8   Roll up through your pelvis to your last rib, then
roll all the way back to rest your pelvis on the floor.
Your pelvis will come away from the floor, but avoid
thrusting it forward; let it hang and only come away
from the floor as much as it needs to. Imagine the
five lumbar bones of your lower back lifting away
from the floor and rolling back down again. Do this
a few times and sense how you roll through your
bones. Rest.

9   Slide your legs away from you, one at a time, and lie
with your legs and arms long. Notice how the curves
of your spine have changed: where does your pelvis
rest now?

10 Bend your knees again, place your feet on the floor
and roll your pelvis slowly away from the floor up to
where you imagine the bottom tips of your shoulder
blades are. Then slowly roll back through your ribs,
lower back, top of the pelvis, sacrum, and tailbone
until your pelvis rests on the floor again. Do this a
few times and see if you can sense every bone lifting
away from the floor and coming back down on the
floor. Come to rest.

11 Now roll your pelvis all the way up to the top of
your shoulder blades. Be sure to stay on top of your

shoulder blades, where they feel broad, and not on your neck. Roll all the way down, bone by bone by bone.

12 Come to rest, slide your legs away one at a time and let yourself completely release on the floor. Notice what you feel and how you feel. Notice the change in your contact with the floor. How are you breathing? What are you thinking?

Ribbon breath

If you find yourself moving into a protected state when you feel anxious or overwhelmed, the first thing to do—presuming that you are not in immediate danger—is to interrupt that process. Try this lesson to stop that thought.

1 Imagine an awareness ribbon: you are going to draw your finger around an imaginary ribbon shape on

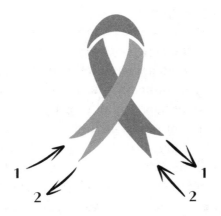

Ribbon breath

the front of your thigh or on your chest, or even on the table in front of you.

2   Start from the left end of the ribbon. As you breathe in, draw your finger from the left bottom to the top of the ribbon; as you breathe out, trace your finger from the top to the bottom right end. Then, as you breathe in again, trace your finger from the right end to the top; as you exhale, trace your finger from the top down to the left end. That makes one round.

3   Repeat for eight rounds, ending with an exhale on the left end of the ribbon.

Self-hug

I use this self-hug to reset my head, neck, and shoulders after a bout of intense focus or being in a fixed position.

1   Come to lie on the floor, with your arms and legs long. Notice how you lie on the floor, what you feel and where you feel it.

2   Now bend your knees and place your feet on the floor. Take the fingers of your right hand under your left armpit, and your left hand onto your right shoulder. Let your elbows rest down gently.

3   Use your right hand to roll your left shoulder blade a small amount to the left, and use your left hand to roll your right shoulder blade a little to the right. Your hands take the weight of your shoulder blades to roll them in the opposite direction, and you are rolling across your back and ribs. Your pelvis is relatively quiet and your knees stay upright; you are

not swaying them wildly from side to side. Don't hold yourself rigid.

4 Rest and let your arms lie by your sides and your legs slide away, one at a time. Notice what you feel now, and how your contact with the floor is different.

5 Bend your knees and place your feet on the floor again. Come back to the same configuration, with your right hand under your left armpit and your left hand on your right shoulder. Come back to rolling your upper and mid-back on the floor, using your hands to pull the shoulder blades in one direction and then the other. Let your head roll with your shoulders, allowing your head to respond to them rolling from one side to the other. Avoid actively rolling your head; it should feel heavy, like a bowling ball. Do this a few times. Notice how your eyeballs roll in your sockets.

6 Rest with your arms by your sides.

7 Bring your arms back to the same configuration and start rolling again, using your hands, but this time rolling your head in opposition to your shoulders. Keep it small and slow and notice how that feels.

8 Rest and let your arms and legs come down by your sides. How do you make contact with the floor now?

9 Repeat this sequence with your left hand under your right armpit, and your right hand on top of your left shoulder.

Here's a simpler variation of this lesson when you need reassurance and grounding:

1 Sit on your sit bones.
2 Place the fingers of your right hand underneath your left armpit, and your left hand on your right shoulder. This stance, with your right hand over the left side of your chest, allows you to feel your heart beating and at the same time gives you a reassuring hold.
3 Breathe in this position, making your exhale longer than your inhale by breathing in for a count of six and exhaling for a count of eight.

Physiological sigh to quickly reduce your stress levels

In this lesson you practice a double inhale through your nose and then you breathe out through your mouth.

1 Breathe in through your nose, then sniff a little bit more air into your nose.
2 Now open your mouth to breathe out.
3 Repeat this three times.

The strategies given above will help you to resolve issues in many different scenarios. Remember to sense what you feel, and to locate yourself in space and time. Soothe your nervous system by giving it reassurance concerning your location in space—be it with your back on the floor, your feet on the floor, your hand on your chest, your sit bones on a chair, or your back against a wall. Tune in to the present moment by feeling the sensations of breathing in and out.

Conclusion

When sleeping women wake, mountains move.
Chinese proverb

Congratulations on reaching the end of the book! You now better understand yourself and how you function, and you can better tune in to your body's sensations.

How are you feeling right now? Take a moment to pause and connect with your body. Notice your breath, your heartbeat, and the tension in your muscles. What does your body have to say to you?

The experience of being in your body is the primary condition of being alive. Yet we often spend our lives hating parts of our bodies, punishing them or noticing only the pain or discomfort. Instead we could feel connected, full of wonder and reverence, and we could attune ourselves to a profound sense of belonging.

The modern world encourages us to outsource our ability to regulate our system. We buy things to make ourselves feel better. We follow fads. We try to think positively. But these things don't always work and can make us feel worse in the long run.

Soothe offers a different approach. It's an *interoceptive* approach, which teaches you to pay attention to your body's sensations and use them to regulate your emotions.

When you learn to listen to your body, you can make informed decisions about what you need to do to feel better.

Cognition happens with your whole self, not just with your mind. Your integrated mind and body are influenced by many factors, including your environment, your circumstances, the suffering of others, and the planet that we all live on. While you can't control the ever-changing environment, you can control how you respond.

The problem with our fast-paced world is that it is full of natural and perceived threats, triggering our "go" mode nervous system into action (see page 34). This can make us feel stuck in a hypervigilant state of restlessness, which may tip over into chronic fatigue and emotional exhaustion. We collectively live through the chaos of the world and are still expected to continue business as usual. How do we hold all of these conflicting states without breaking? The residue of living in a perpetual state of cognitive dissonance takes its toll on the body and brain.

Your superpower is your attention. Paying attention is an effective way to be in an intimate relationship with your life. Learning to soothe starts with learning to feel, which begins with sensing what is happening physically in our bodies. We begin to tune in to the signals that our bodies give us. By gently exploring the flow of the forces through us and by feeling the ground, gravity, and space received by our biointelligent body, we can start to understand that awareness calms the nervous system and encourages better functioning of our soft tissues and organs. By yielding and rocking, we can find a place to unwind our bodies and minds. Our new whole-body organization allows us to embrace our humanness rather than deny it.

This connection enables us to care more deeply for ourselves, live attuned to the rhythm of our bio-intelligent bodies, and be in better relationships with others and with the planet. When you live authentically, you allow other people to feel less alone. When you learn to self-regulate, you also regulate other people around you. We are all interconnected organisms of possibility, connecting with other interconnected organisms of possibility. Everyone I teach—no matter their age, race, socioeconomic status, or circumstances—yearns to be more intimate with their life. You are not stuck, nor are you broken. You have the potential to change and adapt to your ever-changing environment. All you have to do is pause, consider, reorganize, and then decide on the appropriate course of action.

I hope you now understand how you can stay curious and playful, with simple, consistent practices to get interested in the process of living.

All you need to do is to start—one small, soothing step at a time.

Acknowledgments

This book couldn't have been written without a good team helping me to hone and refine. Writing books, it turns out, is quite the challenge.

Thank you to my agent, Valeria, for believing in the book. To all at Profile Books, but especially Cindy, who helped to shape the words by asking me to dig deeper. Cindy's enthusiastic initial response was so encouraging and supportive that I couldn't have published my first book with anyone else.

Thank you to Mandy Greenfield for copyediting, to Holly Kyte for proofreading, and to Emily Frisella at Profile for managing the process.

Thank you to Penguin Life and my US publishing team, including my editor Nina Rodríguez-Marty, publicists Kristina Fazzalaro and Magdalena Deniz, and marketer Chantal Canales. For the cover design, a big thank-you goes to Jason Ramirez, and for copyediting, to Megan Gerrity.

Thank you to all the good people around me who have championed me throughout my evolution from exhausted studio owner to practitioner. In particular, to David Pearl, who has supported me in so many ways, even buying me a laptop when mine crashed in the middle of the first draft, you have been a dear friend to me.

To Georgie Wolfinden from The Beam Room, who has championed me and promoted me during challenging times, and who remained agile even when I changed direction, decided to sell the studios and move to the sea, and reinvented myself as a Somatic

Movement Educator along the way (while going through menopause and then the pandemic).

Thank you to Susan Riley, who has helped me to make shape of my ideas over the years. To Farrah Storr, for supporting me through my many evolutions and helping me to brainstorm ideas for The Human Method, and who got me onto Substack, where my newsletter lives. To Lucie Seffens for championing me. To Rebecca Newman for letting me sound out a few ideas. To the lovely Kirsty Wallace and Luella, who sent me care packages and cards throughout the writing process and were the first people to read the introduction of my book.

And thanks to all my friends who have listened to me talking about my book for such a long time.

Thank you to everyone in the wellness and beauty world who has shown interest in my work and given me a platform, in particular to Ateh Jewel for her generous heart.

I would be nothing without brilliant teachers and teaching over the years, so thank you to Garet Newell, Director of the Feldenkrais Training Centre in the UK, for your passionate teaching and for bringing the Feldenkrais Method to the UK. To Judith Hanson Lasseter, for your compassionate teaching; to Gary Carter, for his nondogmatic and awe-inspiring teaching; to Michael Stone, for his vulnerable tenderness and humor. And to Ben Wolff, for his sharp ability to get to the nub of things, thank you for shining the light. Thank you to the inspiring teachers whose work has helped and influenced me: Stephen Batchelor, Dr. Richard Brown, and Dr. Patricia Gerberg; the work of Ruthy Alon, Bonnie Bainbridge Cohen, David Zemach-Bersin, and Jeff Haller; and to the Somatic Yoga and Feldenkrais community in the UK Internationally.

Thank you to all my clients, who sharpen my skills every time we meet in online classes, private sessions, courses, and in person on retreats and workshops.

A special mention to Sarah Brooks who has encouraged and supported me to do bold things over the years. And to Caroline Banks who kindly champions me.

Thank you to everyone who supports my work on Substack, including the founding members.

Thank you to my mum for showing me how to be fearless, and in memory of my dad, who boldly made a life for us all in London. I wish he knew that I wrote a book.

Thank you again to Rudy, my clever and compassionate husband, who cooked for me, edited the first drafts, took the dogs out for walks, and fully lived through the process. Life wouldn't be half as fun without him by my side.

Last of all thank you to my dogs, Lucky Pierre, Bon Bon, and Lil' Louis for showing me how to tend to your nervous system with sleep, running, rolling, and play.

Notes

1 Your Body

1 Vandana Shiva is an environmental activist, food-sovereignty advocate, ecofeminist, and anti-globalization author.
2 René Descartes, *Meditations on First Philosophy* (1641).
3 Dr. Susan Greenfield, *A Day in the Life of the Brain: The Neuroscience of Consciousness from Dawn Till Dusk* (Allen Lane, 2016).
4 Moshe Feldenkrais, *Awareness Through Movement* (Thorsons, 1991).
5 Lisa Feldman Barrett, *How Emotions Are Made* (Macmillan, 2017).
6 Ibid.
7 Ibid.
8 Martin P. Paulus and Murray B. Stein, "Interoception in anxiety and depression," *Brain Structure & Function*, 214(5), (2010), www.ncbi.nlm.nih.gov/pmc/articles/PMC2886901/.
9 Dr. Bessel van der Kolk, *The Body Keeps the Score: Mind, Brain and Body in the Healing of Trauma* (Viking, 2014).
10 Linda Hartley, *Wisdom of the Body Moving* (North Atlantic Books, 1995).

2 Body Sensing

1 Van der Kolk, *The Body Keeps the Score*.
2 Ibid.
3 Feldman Barrett, *How Emotions Are Made*.
4 Russell Foster, *Life Time: The New Science of the Body Clock,*

and How It Can Revolutionize Your Sleep and Health (Penguin Life, 2022).

5   Lisa Feldman Barrett, *Seven and a Half Lessons About the Brain* (Picador, 2021).

6   Scientists don't seem to have a consensus on the terms used to describe the flow of information from your body to your brain. So that I am clear throughout the book, I use these terms to convey specific meanings. "Embodiment" is the experience of being a physical body in the world; it is the awareness of our own bodies and the sensations that we feel in them. Embodiment also includes the ability to control our bodies and move through the world. "Somatic awareness" is the specific awareness of our bodily sensations—the ability to pay attention to the way our bodies feel, both in the moment and over time.

7   *The Science of Vision, Eye Health & Seeing Better*, Huberman Lab podcast, episode 24.

8   "Research: US adults spend 44 years staring at screens," Advanced Television, June 4, 2020, https://advanced-television .com/2020/06/04/research-us-adults-spend-44-years-staring -at-screens/.

9   Justin C. Sherwin et al., "The association between time spent outdoors and myopia in children and adolescents: a systematic review and meta-analysis," *Ophthalmology*, 119(10), (October 2012), pubmed.ncbi.nlm.nih.gov/22809757/.

10   Rose Eveleth, *How do we smell?* TED-Ed, www.youtube.com/ watch?v=snJnO6OpjCs.

11   *How Smell, Taste & Pheromone-Like Chemicals Control You*, Huberman Lab podcast, episode 25.

12   Nadine Gogolla, "The insular cortex," *Science Direct*, 27(12), (2017), www.sciencedirect.com/science/article/pii/ S0960982217305468.

13   *How to Control Your Sense of Pain & Pleasure*, Huberman Lab podcast, episode 32.

14   Dacher Keltner, "The science of touch: why physical contact can make you happier and more successful," *Wired* (2017), www.wired.co.uk/article/the-good-life-human-touch.

15   Ibid.

16   Feldman Barrett, *How Emotions Are Made.*

3 The Breath

1   Gerhard Whitworth, "Normal Respiratory Rates: Adults and
      Children," MedicalNewsToday, February 11, 2019, https://
      www.medicalnewstoday.com/articles/324409.

2   Jennifer Huizen, "How COVID-19 has changed the face of the
      natural world," *Medical News Today* (22 April 2021), www
      .medicalnewstoday.com/articles/how-covid-19-has-changed-
      the-face-of-the-natural-world#Wildlife-and-COVID-19:-
      The-good.

3   "Understanding the stress response," Harvard Health Publishing
      (6 July 2020), www.health.harvard.edu/staying-healthy/
      understanding-the-stress-response.

4   "You are your brain," Healthy Brains by Cleveland Clinic,
      healthybrains.org/brain-facts/.

5   Roger E. Bohn and James E. Short, "How Much Information?:
      2009 Report on American Consumers," Global Information
      Industry Center (9 December 2009), art2science.files.wordpress
      .com/2009/12/hmi_2009_consumerreport_dec9_2009.pdf.

6   Marcos Domic-Siede, "Emotion regulation strategies and the
      two-dimensional model of adult attachment: a pilot study,"
      Frontiers in Behavioural Neuroscience (7 July 2023), pubmed
      .ncbi.nlm.nih.gov/37484522/.

7   Isnaini Herawati et al., "Breathing exercise for hypertensive
      patients: A scoping review," *Frontiers in Physiology* (25 January
      2023), www.ncbi.nlm.nih.gov/pmc/articles/PMC9905130/.

8   J. Yesmin, N. Begum and S. Ferdousi, "Effect of Slow Breathing
      Exercise on Glycaemic Status in Type 2 Diabetic Male
      Patients," *Mymensingh Medical Journal*, 31(1), (January 2022),
      pubmed.ncbi.nlm.nih.gov/34999707/.

9   Jungwon Min et al., "Modulating heart rate oscillation affects
      plasma amyloid beta and tau levels in younger and older
      adults," *Scientific Reports*, 13 (9 March 2023), www.nature
      .com/articles/s41598-023-30167-0.

10 Stephen Elliott, *The New Science of Breath* (Coherence Publishing, 2005).

11 Brenda Carla Lima Araújo et al., "Association Between Mouth Breathing and Asthma: a Systematic Review and Meta-analysis," *Current Allergy and Asthma Reports*, 20(7), (19 May 2020), pubmed.ncbi.nlm.nih.gov/32430704/; Vincent Yi-Fong Su et al., "Mouth opening/breathing is common in sleep apnea and linked to more nocturnal water loss," *Biomedical Journal*, 46(3), (June 2023), www.ncbi.nlm.nih.gov/pmc/articles/PMC10209680/.

12 In 2017 *Frontiers in Psychology* found that people who practiced slow breathing for twenty minutes a day for four weeks had a significant reduction in stress levels, as measured by the Perceived Stress Scale (PSS). The study also found that slow breathing improved sleep quality and reduced blood pressure. And in 2018 *Biological Psychology* found that slow breathing improved focus and attention in healthy adults. The study participants who practiced slow breathing for twenty minutes a day for four weeks showed significant improvements in a task that required them to focus on a small target while ignoring distractions.

13 Richard P. Brown and Patricia L. Gerbarg, *The Healing Power of the Breath* (Trumpeter Books, 2012).

14 Susan I. Hopper et al., "Effectiveness of diaphragmatic breathing for reducing physiological and psychological stress in adults: a quantitative systematic review," *JBI Database of Systematic Reviews and Implementation Reports*, 17(9), (September 2019), pubmed.ncbi.nlm.nih.gov/31436595/; Kevin Gipson et al., "Sleep-Disordered Breathing in Children," *Paediatric Review*, 40(1), (January 2019), www.ncbi.nlm.nih.gov/pmc/articles/PMC6557418/; Robin E. Cushing and Kathryn L. Braun, "Mind-Body Therapy for Military Veterans with Post-Traumatic Stress Disorder: A Systematic Review," *Journal of Alternative and Complementary Medicine*, 23(2), (February 2019), pubmed.ncbi.nlm.nih.gov/28880607/.

4 Touch

1   Gabor Maté, *Hold On to Your Kids: Why Parents Need to Matter More Than Peers* (Ballantine Books, 2005).

2   Ashley Montagu, *Touching: The Human Significance of the Skin* (Columbia University Press, 1971).

3   Francis McGlone and Susannah Walker, "Four health benefits of hugs—and why they feel so good," *The Conversation* (17 May 2021).

4   "Touch—the Forgotten Sense with Professor Francis McGlone," *Feel Better, Live More with Dr. Rangan Chatterjee*, episode 45 (16 January 2019).

5   Montagu, *Touching: The Human Significance of the Skin.*

6   McGlone and Walker, "Four health benefits of hugs."

7   Karen M. Grewen et al., "Warm partner contact is related to lower cardiovascular reactivity," *Behavioral Medicine*, 29(3), (2003), pubmed.ncbi.nlm.nih.gov/15206831/.

5 Move

1   Moshé Feldenkrais was a biophysicist, mechanical engineer and self-taught educator who developed a method of movement education called the Feldenkrais Method. He was born in 1904 in what is now Ukraine and emigrated to Israel in 1954. The Feldenkrais Method is based on the idea that the brain and body are inseparable. It uses gentle movements and verbal cues to help people improve their movement patterns and develop greater awareness of their bodies.

2   "Mind-body connection is built into brain: Findings point to brain areas that integrate planning, purpose, physiology, behavior, movement," Washington University School of Medicine, *Science Daily* (19 April 2023), www.sciencedaily.com/releases/2023/04/230419125052.htm.

3   "Exercise linked to improved mental health, but more may not always be better," *The Lancet* (8 August 2018), www.sciencedaily.com/releases/2018/08/180808193656.htm.

4   "Physical Activity, Fitness, and Physical Education: Effects on

Academic Performance," *Educating the Student Body: Taking Physical Activity and Physical Education to School* (National Academies Press, 2013).

5 J. Eric Ahlskog et al., "Physical Exercise as a Preventive or Disease-Modifying Treatment of Dementia and Brain Aging," *Mayo Clinic Proceedings*, 86(9), (September 2011), www.ncbi .nlm.nih.gov/pmc/articles/PMC3258000/.

6 Kelly McGonigal, *The Upside of Stress: Why Stress Is Good for You and How to Get Good at It* (Avery Publishing, 2015).

7 Abiola Keller et al., "Does the perception that stress affects health matter? The association with health and mortality," *Health Psychology*, 31(5), (September 2012), pubmed.ncbi.nlm .nih.gov/22201278/.

8 "Understanding the stress response," Harvard Health Publishing (6 July 2020), www.health.harvard.edu/staying-healthy/ understanding-the-stress-response.

9 Hans Selye, *The Stress of Life* (revised and expanded edition 1982).

6 Rest

1 In her book *Letter to My Daughter* (Random House, 2008), Angelou writes about the importance of taking time for oneself, even when life is busy and stressful.

2 Coined by Andrew Huberman—a nondogmatic term to refer to body-sensing meditation.

3 Jack Flynn, "20 Incredible Productivity Statistics [2022]: Average Employee Productivity in the U.S.," Zippia, November 2, 2022, https://www.zippia.com/advice/productivity-statistics/.

4 Jeff Rumage, "Presenteeism: Definition, Causes, Consequences," Built In, https://builtin.com/employee-engagement/ presenteeism.

5 The four-day workweek trial in the UK was organized by 4 Day Week Global, a nonprofit organization that advocates a shorter working week. The trial was funded by the Joseph Rowntree Foundation, a charitable organization that supports social change.

6   K. Anders Ericsson, Ralf T. Krampe, and Clemens Tesch-Römer, "The role of deliberate practice in the acquisition of expert performance," *Psychological Review*, 100(3), (1993), psycnet .apa.org/record/1993-40718-001.

7   Alex Soojung-Kim Pang, *Rest: Why You Get More Done When You Work Less* (Basic Books, 2016).

8   Ryan Fiorenzi, "Sleep Statistics: Understanding Sleep and Sleep Disorders," Start Sleeping, 2019, https://startsleeping.org/ statistics/.

7 Nourishment

1   Michael Pollan, *In Defense of Food: An Eater's Manifesto* (Allen Lane, 2008). Pollan is an American author and journalist who writes about food, agriculture, and the environment.

2   "Fast Food Restaurants in the US—Market Size, Industry Analysis, Trends and Forecasts (2024–2029)," Ibis World, October 2023, https://www.ibisworld.com/united-states/market -research-reports/fast-food-restaurants-industry/#IndustryStati sticsAndTrends.

3   Evelyn Medawar et al., "The effects of plant-based diets on the body and the brain: a systematic review," *Transactional Psychiatry*, 9 (12 September 2109), www.nature.com/articles/ s41398-019-0552-0.

4   Robert K. McNamara and Susan E. Carlson, "Role of omega-3 fatty acids in brain development and function," *Prostaglandins, Leukotrienes & Essential Fatty Acids*, 75(4–5), (2006), pubmed .ncbi.nlm.nih.gov/16949263/.

5   Athena Enderami et al., "The effects and potential mechanisms of folic acid on cognitive function: a comprehensive review," *Neurological Science*, 39(10), (October 2018), pubmed.ncbi .nlm.nih.gov/29936555/.

6   Health Quality Ontario, "Vitamin B12 and cognitive function: an evidence-based analysis," Ontario Health Technology Assessment Series, 13(23), (1 November 2103), pubmed.ncbi .nlm.nih.gov/24379897.

7   Ignacio Jáuregui-Lobera, "Iron deficiency and cognitive
    functions," *Neuropsychiatric Disease and Treatment* 10 (2014),
    www.ncbi.nlm.nih.gov/pmc/articles/PMC4235202/.
8   Grace A. Ogunrinola et al., "The Human Microbiome and Its
    Impacts on Health," *International Journal of Microbiology*,
    v.2020 (2020), www.ncbi.nlm.nih.gov/pmc/articles/
    PMC7306068/.
9   "The SMILES trial," Food & Mood Centre, Deakin University,
    foodandmoodcentre.com.au/smiles-trial/.
10 Emeran A. Mayer et al., "The Gut–Brain Axis," *Annual Review
    of Medicine*, 73 (27 January 2022), pubmed.ncbi.nlm.nih
    .gov/34669431/. Timothy G. Dinan and John F. Cryan, "Gut
    instincts: microbiota as a key regulator of brain development,
    ageing and neurodegeneration," *Journal of Physiology*,
    595(2), (15 January 2017), www.ncbi.nlm.nih.gov/pmc/articles/
    PMC5233671/.
11 Mireia Gascon et al., "Residential green spaces and mortality:
    A systematic review," *Environment International*, 86 (January
    2016), pubmed.ncbi.nlm.nih.gov/26540085/.
12 Ming Kuo, "How might contact with nature promote human
    health? Promising mechanisms and a possible central pathway,"
    Frontiers in Psychology, 6 (25 August 2015), www.frontiersin
    .org/articles/10.3389/fpsyg.2015.01093/full.

8 Connect

1   As well as being a Buddhist monk, Jack Kornfield is a
    clinical psychologist and mindfulness teacher. He introduced
    mindfulness practice to the West and has written sixteen books.
2   Paul D. MacLean, *The Triune Brain in Evolution* (Springer,
    1990).
3   Brian Dean, "167 Incredible Digital Marketing Stats,"
    Backlinko, last updated January 26, 2021, https://backlinko
    .com/digital-marketing-stats.
4   Brian Dean, "133 Super Interesting Social Marketing Media
    Stats," Backlinko, last updated August 18, 2023, https://
    backlinko.com/social-media-marketing-stats.

5 Rob Binns, "Screen time statistics 2024: Global increases/ decreases, mobile vs desktop, and screen time's effects on children," Independent Advisor, last updated September 5, 2023, https://www.independent.co.uk/advisor/vpn/ screen-time-statistics.

6 Joenna Driemeyer et al., "Changes in Gray Matter Induced by Learning—Revisited," PLoS One, 3(7), (2008), www.ncbi.nlm .nih.gov/pmc/articles/PMC2447176/.

7 Sy Atezaz Saeed et al., "Exercise, yoga, and meditation for depressive and anxiety disorders," American Family Physician (15 April 2010), pubmed.ncbi.nlm.nih.gov/20387774/.

8 M. D. Fox, M. E. Raichle and K. Christoff, "The default mode network: A system for social cognition and internal thought," Trends in Cognitive Sciences, 9(6), (2005).

9 "Fashion brands failing to pay living wages to garment workers," Fashion Checker (2020).

10 P. Smith, "Revenue of the apparel market worldwide by country in 2023," February 9, 2024, https://www.statista.com /forecasts/758683/revenue-of-the-apparel-market-worldwide -by-country.

9 The Principles of The Soothe Program

1 Jiddu Krishnamurti, Think on These Things (1964). Krishnamurti is considered one of the greatest philosophers and teachers of all time, his work influencing major figures such as George Bernard Shaw, David Bohm, Alan Watts, Henry Miller, Bruce Lee, Jackson Pollock, and Aldous Huxley.

Index